I0463845

FORTY-FIVE
YEARS IN WHITE UNIFORMS

FORTY-FIVE
YEARS IN WHITE UNIFORMS

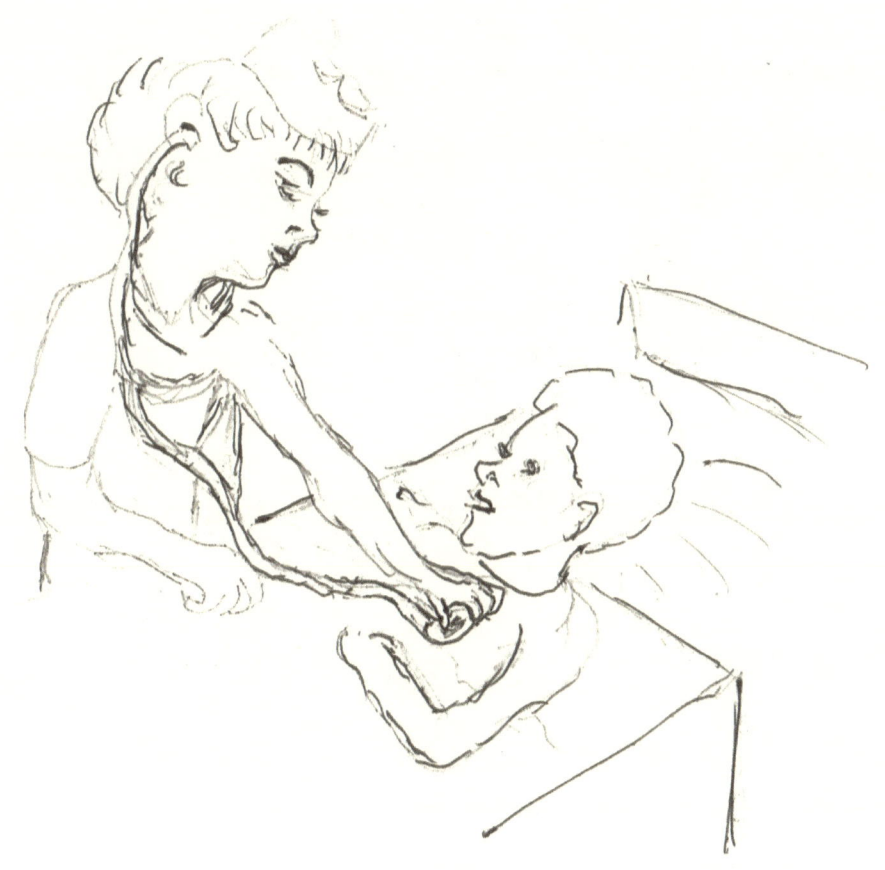

C.L.G. SOLOMON

Copyright © 2013 by C.L.G. Solomon.

Library of Congress Control Number:		2013911136
ISBN:	Hardcover	978-1-4836-5648-9
	Softcover	978-1-4836-5647-2
	Ebook	978-1-4836-5649-6

All rights reserved. No part of this book may be reproduced or transmitted in any form or by any means, electronic or mechanical, including photocopying, recording, or by any information storage and retrieval system, without permission in writing from the copyright owner.

This book was printed in the United States of America.

Rev. date: 06/21/2013

To order additional copies of this book, contact:
Xlibris Corporation
1-888-795-4274
www.Xlibris.com
Orders@Xlibris.com
130970

Contents

*"Lives of great men all remind us
We can make our lives sublime,
And, departing, leave behind us
Footprints in the sands of time."*

—*Henry Wadsworth Longfellow*

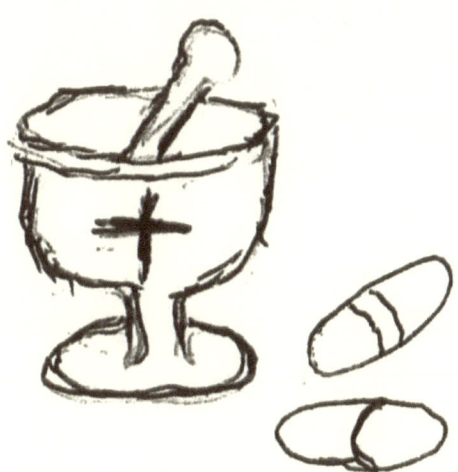

Stay healthy

Introduction

Forty five years in white uniforms

From the pen of the same writer of the book *Natural Bread Is Not Enough* comes a partial biographical account of her forty-five-year nursing career. Seventeen years were spent working in various disciplines of nursing, while the final twenty-eight years were spent working in public health nursing.

In keeping with HIPPA laws, which are designed to protect the privacy of clients and their information, no part of this writing at any point ever divulges anyone's name or records. The information is recollected from various work experiences, in various cities and states, over a period of years.

Forty-five years have not qualified me to be an authority in the nursing field. It has simply given me various insights that someone else may read about and make a quality career decision. I had classmates who dropped out of nursing school and stated, "Nursing definitely is not for me."

Some students failed because they underestimated the amount of study and dedication involved in becoming a nurse. Some students were not willing to spend long hours in study and research. Some found that the sights and smells of blood and other body fluids were definite turnoffs.

One other classmate completed the entire nursing program with a 4.0 average, only to say she hated it. She never practiced a day of nursing. She excelled in clinicals as well as in the classroom. She received the highest academic award in our class, yet nursing was not her cup of tea.

The experiences that I encountered in my personal life somewhat intensified my desire to become a nurse. I am happy to have been able to practice the kind of work that was very satisfying to me. The nursing knowledge that paralleled certain difficult times in my life was priceless.

Nursing is the type of profession that one can practice in different settings with various categories of people, such as the aged, the middle aged, the young adults, the teens, the expectant moms and their children—the newborn, premature babies—and people with special needs.

Work settings run the gamut from hospitals to jails, institutions, the military, private homes, clinics, schools, rehabilitation centers of different types, and other settings not mentioned. Someone once said, "Variety is the spice of life." Variety abounds in the nursing profession.

A nurse can expand on her career by becoming an advanced registered nurse practitioner, nurse anesthetist, midwife, legal consultant, or she may go on to medical school to be a physician. Nurses also train other nurses. Administration is another career option within nursing.

One of the first things a prospective nurse needs to consider is which type of program she should choose. Some students choose the certified nursing assistant (CNA) program. They want to obtain some of the basic skills and a quick job. These skills often include learning to take vital signs, such as blood pressure, pulse, and respiration.

They learn how to do basic care and other skills that can assist the nurse in his/her work. CNA skills can serve as a pivotal point for the person to move higher into the medical profession. Some certified nursing assistants advance their training and become registered nurses and doctors.

Nurses are trained in programs of different length and at different levels. Licensed practical nurses, or LPNS, may train one or more years depending on where they train. Registered nurses, or RNs, may complete an associate's degree and start work after licensure. RNs may also complete a four-year baccalaureate-degree program. All levels must be certified.

Some medical facilities offer CNA training whereby a student may work and train in their facility at the same time. Upon completion of training, the student is expected to work for the institution for a contracted amount of time. The student may stop at this level or move further into the profession.

Associate and baccalaureate programs are located on College campuses. A College degree is earned at these schools. All level nurses must obtain clinical experiences in a medical institution. Clinical experiences usually consist of medical, surgical, psychiatric, pediatric, and maternal and child health.

During my years at the associate's degree College, initial training was focused on obtaining College math, arts, sciences, chemistry, anatomy and physiology, psychology, communications, and human growth and development. Caregiving skills may be concurrent with academic work.

Before many of the specialized programs came into being, nurses were required to draw blood, perform respiratory therapy skills, assist in delivering babies, and perform whatever other tasks got the job done. The advent of the special programs has freed nurses to focus on nursing.

During my baccalaureate training, the main focus, in addition to learning technical skills, was the scientific principles of why we did what we did. Information tends to be remembered better if the rationale is known for what you are doing.

Nurses must pass a state examination to be licensed. Strengthen your studies in math, science, and communications. Working as a volunteer can also give you some insight into what the medical profession is all about. New short-term nursing programs have emerged, which should ease the projected shortages.

Nursing is not a profession that lends itself to boredom because its areas are so varied. It is like having the option to work different jobs within one profession. In this era in which we live, nurses remain very much in demand. There are even nurse recruiters.

Various portions of this writing will contain scriptures wherever they are applicable. When dealing with the events of life and death, scripture seems to have a place. Nursing is a life-and-death-related occupation. Chaplains are hired to attend to the spiritual needs of patients in medical institutions.

After studying and reading scriptures for so long a time in my life, they have become a part of me. The Holy Spirit brings other scriptures to mind as I am writing. Many who read my first book told me they enjoyed and were inspired by those scriptures.

When I stick with the word, it gives illumination to my life and light to my path. I never understood what "Rhema word" meant until prior to writing my first book. That is when the Holy Spirit really reveals the meaning of a scripture to you. This happened during the writing of my first book.

Living within the guidelines of the Word is like having a built-in compass. In the absence of consistent role models, the Word provides powerful guidance. Some patients are comforted when they know their caregivers are guided by the Lord.

When nurses complete their training, they must go before a licensure board. They must be licensed in the state in which they plan to practice. Nurses can practice in other states with their own state license, provided the other state has what is known as reciprocity.

Usually government institutions allow practitioners holding any state nursing license to practice in them. Upon successful completion of the state nursing examination, nurses are issued a license. Continuing education units must be obtained every two years for license renewal.

Licensure ensures the minimum standard of a safe practitioner. Medical institutions require that new practitioners go through orientation programs.

The programs allow the institution to assess the new employees' knowledge base and skill levels.

Safe practice is stressed because the business of dealing with people's lives is crucial. Humans can perform CPR, but they cannot replace carelessly lost lives. Only those serious about human life should consider a medical career. Fragile lives such as babies and the elderly can easily ebb away under the hands of careless, unsafe practitioners.

While the nursing profession is an enjoyable career for many, it requires diligence, knowledge, skill, vigilance, endurance, tact, and wisdom. Autonomy and ability to follow instructions are must-haves. Compassion and/or empathy must be possessed qualities to reach the souls of people.

Lady with the lamp

When one begins to talk about the events of nursing, its founder, Florence Nightingale, has to be remembered. This work will not attempt to present a lengthy discourse on Ms. Nightingale's life and her accomplishments. Much is already written, and some of the references are included at the end of this book.

Our initial nursing history classes introduced us to our nursing pioneer, Florence Nightingale. She forged a path through history that set the stage for today's practice ethics. There were other pioneers in nursing, but she was the major pioneer. Her efforts were most outstanding. Although she has been harshly criticized by some, her good works prevail.

Ms. Nightingale was born on May 12, 1820, in Florence, Italy. She died on August 13, 1910, in London, United Kingdom. Her life and career spanned ninety years, when many people did not survive long life spans. She is an excellent example of one having dreams, goals, and purposes to live.

Even Florence Nightingale's nursing endeavors were inspired by her desire to fulfill what she felt was a God-given call on her life. She felt that relieving the sick and suffering was her mission in life. She had a vision, and she fulfilled it. She left guidelines that are applicable in today's society.

Although there have been nursing acts since biblical times and nurses are mentioned in the Bible, Ms. Nightingale is the person who caused nursing to be recognized as an organized profession. Nursing acts of biblical times will be addressed briefly at some point in this work.

Ms. Nightingale had the foresight to become involved in the political system also. While politics are often painted as undesirable, much has been accomplished when channeled by way of the political system. Prayer is a powerful force, yet legislation brought about changes that were not wanted by everyone on the subject of prayer.

As a result of Ms. Nightingale's political efforts and foresight, much was accomplished in bringing nursing into the forefront. The nursing profession today has, as its bargaining force, the American Nurses Association. Each state and city has its own nursing association chapter.

While these groups seem relatively quiet and not always widely known, they wield much power in accomplishing changes that need to take place within the profession. Some of the chapters have lobbyists who attend political sessions, and they make strides as needed within the profession.

During my nursing days, a group of us traveled to Tallahassee, Florida, the state's capital, to lobby on an issue. Lobbying goes on all the time, either for or against issues. The people who stay on top of issues usually win. Every vote counts in every election of any kind.

The system of government touches much of our lives; thus we need to be at least familiar with its workings. Because nursing is an ever-evolving profession, nurses need to be in positions where we can affect positive change. Colleges also have and encourage student nursing chapter participation.

Being wealthy, well educated, brilliant, astute, well traveled, and well known gave Ms. Nightingale the advantages she needed. She was able to activate political, social, and statistical reforms in the profession. These reforms are responsible for some of the progress we enjoy in the profession.

Florence Nightingale was responsible for many reforms in medical institutions. She saw firsthand the results of care with unwashed hands. The importance of hand washing and cleanliness in enhancing healing was one of her most notable contributions to the health profession.

Standards continue to exist today that ensure safe care for the sick and suffering. All practitioners are required to meet certain standards before entering the profession. Those who violate the codes and standards are ousted from the profession. Incarceration is also a possible consequence.

Florence Nightingale saw the need for nurses to be trained, so she opened one of the first nursing schools. St. Thomas Hospital of London, England, was the site of the school. She received many meritorious awards and honors for her work in improving the status of those who were suffering.

Florence lived in an era where medical conditions were deplorable. Her nursing work in the Crimean War, which was fought between Britain and Russia in 1854, and her work in the Barrack Hospital of Uskudar in Anatolia, Turkey, gave her deep insight into the problems of caring for the sick.

During my hospital working days, we complained about the lack of supplies. Shiploads of supplies sank in the icy waters during Florence's era, forcing staff to work with nothing. They worked against odds that we can never imagine. Death and infection were constant stalkers in the bitter cold.

Ms. Nightingale had one older sister. Florence never married nor birthed any children. History has it that she turned down a longtime admirer, choosing instead to devote her life to her calling of relieving human suffering.

Florence Nightingale was affectionately known as the Lady with the Lamp. She could be seen walking the long and dark halls at the military hospital, carrying her lamp in her quest to relieve the wounded, suffering, and dying. All reading references about Florence are highly recommended.

Nursing attire

The title *Forty-Five Years in White Uniforms* refers to the extinct practice of nurses being decked out in all-white attire. For many years, I headed to work in a white uniform, white hose, white oxford shoes, and a white cap. This attire identified all wearers as nurses.

Caps were worn to keep the nurse's hair in place and to give her a modest appearance. There were also concerns that loose-flowing hair could present a health hazard by getting into the clients' face, the work surface, or any open wounds. Hair was also contained in a net or with hair spray.

Nursing caps once set female nurses apart from other staff. The practice of wearing caps is rarely seen. Caps were recently thought to be fomites. Fomites are objects that absorb and transmit infectious material. Nurses' caps were originally worn at the beginning of a nurse's clinical training.

Capping ceremonies were once one of the highlights of the student nurses' training. Each school had its own particular cap design. Caps were worn in Florence Nightingale's time. Caps may be seen more in developing nations than in the United States. Caps may also be worn more by nurses in smaller towns.

Nursing pins continue to be a part of many nurses' attire. Nurses looked forward to the day when they would receive their pin. Pinning ceremonies, which officially welcomed nurses into the profession, took place near graduation. Pins and caps identified one's alma mater.

Every nurse wore a watch with the sweep second hand for checking pulses and respirations. All medical personnel still wear such watches. Name tags were worn and are still worn for identification. Makeup was to be very light, again to appear modest.

Today's nurse blends with everyone else. Many wear scrub suits of varied colors or prints. Lab coats are worn by many types of medical staff, so nurses are not easily identified anymore. Various departments may only be identified among each other by the color of their scrubs.

Even students are barely identifiable. If they are carrying books or are traveling in groups, it may be assumed that they are students, but not really known. Some nursing staff members wear casual clothing under a laboratory coat. Only a close look at someone's name tag may reveal his or her title.

It is not the attire that makes the person. It is that look of compassion, that caring heart, those gentle hands, and tact and diplomacy. Another feature about uniforms was that they struck fear in the hearts of children. Children made an unpleasant association between the white attire and the nurse.

Some kids started screaming when the wearer of white attire came in their direction. Surely the wearer of the white was bringing a shot or was going to perform some painful procedure. Less of this is seen with the pleasant pastel colors.

ACKNOWLEDGMENTS

My special thanks go to various people. Special thanks to all of my professors from each College I attended. With your help, I was able to obtain my Associate of arts, Bachelor of Science in nursing ed., Master of Arts in theology, Specialist in Christian counseling, and Doctorate of ministry in theology. To one of my baby sisters, thanks for your frequent encouraging phone calls from up North and your raves about my first book. To another baby sister, who recently moved to Pennsylvania, thanks for your loving calls and encouragement. To my brothers and their wives, thanks for your book raves and your encouragement.

Thanks to the rest of my family. You continue to show your love and support in many ways. I love you. To my nieces, nephews, and cousins, you are not forgotten. Auntie loves all of you.

Thanks to all of the hospitals and clinics that gave me jobs during my youthful and productive working years. To both health clinics in different cities, thanks for many happy moments of public health and clinical nursing experiences. I often reflect on the years spent with you.

To Healthy Start, which is a public health program designed to ensure healthy outcomes to pregnant moms and their babies, thanks! You gave me many years of pleasurable work. Administrators and other staff provided some of the most pleasant working environments one could enter.

To the doctor and his nurse who helped me with my first nursing experience, thanks for believing in me. Thanks to one counselor and former classmate from my hometown for your raving review about my book *Natural Bread Is Not Enough*. To all that either prayed for or encouraged me, thanks!

Special thanks to my pastor and minister, his mom, and all members of my church for the past ten years. In addition to your prayers and encouragements, you have provided space for the display of my books. I appreciate all of your acts of kindness and love.

Thanks to Ms. SP, the retired schoolteacher. You have shown your true love as a sister in Christ. You made yourself available to proofread, edit, and provide resources for me this time, just as you did with *Natural Bread Is Not Enough*.

Thanks to my fellow prayer partners throughout the city of my residence. You have continued to bathe me and my efforts in prayer. To the prayer captain and the effectual praying ladies of our prayer ministry. Thanks!

Nurses mentioned in the Word

"And they sent away Rebekah their sister, and her nurse, and Abraham's servant and his men" Genesis 24:59. The occasion was the acquiring of a wife for Isaac, Abraham's son of promise. As Abraham was getting ready to make his earthly departure, he made preparation for a good wife for his son.

Abraham sent his servant among their kinfolk in another city to select Isaac's wife. Abraham knew the importance of selecting a woman who was not of the heathen women in his living area. God had promised and given him a son, now he wanted to preserve the integrity of his progeny by selecting the right mate for Isaac.

Abraham's servant had prayed for God to make his way prosperous in obtaining a bride for his master. The things he asked God to do in order to confirm the choice of a bride for Isaac, God did. As the story goes, Isaac was very pleased with Rebekah and took her as his bride.

Nurses were considered very honorable and important people in Bible days. Rebekah's nurse lived and traveled with her and her family. A considerable amount of time had lapsed in Rebekah's life when her nurse died. "But Deborah, Rebekah's nurse, died, and she was buried beneath Bethel under an oak" Genesis 35:8.

"And Jonathan, Saul's son, had a son that was lame of his feet, and was five years old when the tidings came of Saul and Jonathan out of Jezreel, and his nurse took him up, and fled: and it came to pass, as she made haste to flee, that he fell and became lame. And his name was Mephibosheth" 2 Samuel 4:4.

Saul was the first king anointed and appointed by God over the children of Israel. When the news of Saul's and his son Jonathan's death came, Saul's grandson, Mephibosheth was taken up by his nurse. As they were running, the grandson fell and became lame. The first four chapters of 2 Samuel give the account of the story.

"But a certain Samaritan, as he journeyed, came where he was: and when he saw him, he had compassion on him, and went to him, and bound up his wounds, pouring in oil and wine, and set him on his own beast, and brought him to an inn, and took care of him" Luke 10:33-34.

There was a time when the profession was top-heavy with women. There are now many male nurses. This Samaritan was a male who nursed this man who had fallen among thieves. The thieves had stripped him and wounded him, leaving him half dead. The Good Samaritan helped him. The priest and the Levite passed by and overlooked the wounded man.

MY FOOT STEPS
WERE ORDERED

"Order my steps in thy word, and let not any iniquity have dominion over me" Psalm 119:133. As I reflect over the past forty-five years of my nursing career, I can see and say that my steps were ordered by the Lord. As you read, you may agree with me.

After all, music and art talents are in my heritage. Presently, my older brother, of Ft. Lauderdale, Florida, is exercising his musical talents in the rhythm-and-blues field. He has carved out a world career in his craft. Another cousin, of Macon, Georgia, has spent many years writing and playing music.

Another cousin who dedicated her music career to the Lord is using it to his glory today in the California area. Others have written music and carved out careers in the natural talents passed on to us by our forefathers.

Out of all the gifted ones, my life's turn of events led me into the medical field. While I still love music and art and I dabble in both, my forte has been a career in nursing. Although I took piano and organ lessons, during my youth, I am no virtuoso. Some people claimed to have enjoyed my music playing.

My observations of sickness, suffering, and disadvantageous situations of others influenced my desire to do something about them. I had my own set of hurts that needed nurturing. A career in the medical field seemed to be the vantage point from which to work.

My dad started my siblings and me singing in church. He lined us up across the floor of the old Methodist church and had us singing songs. Our repertoire included songs from the Grand Ole Opry radio show and the songs our mom sang to us in the daytime. I remember singing all of my childhood days.

I enjoyed those times of singing. We gathered around the radio on Saturday nights to practice the songs. Those were our first official voice lessons. The remainder of the week, we spent our time playing out in the vast yard where we lived in the woods. We swung on an old tire swing hanging from a large tree in the backyard.

There were large drums also on the property. I believe they were associated with our dad's work. We rolled each other around in those drums as we played in those carefree days. A group of Caucasian children lived somewhere in the area. Some days they would just show up, and we would swing on the swing and play in our yard.

We never knew where they came from, and we never went to their houses. Nobody asked any questions, and we just played peacefully together. When the children left, we would go inside our house until the next time.

One Sunday, when we returned home from singing, we encountered a couple sitting on our porch. They came to get two of us to live with them. They had heard that a man had some children he was giving away. We didn't know that we were the kids they came to get.

The lady was rocking in her chair. As we drew nearer to the porch, she stopped rocking, leaned forward in her chair, and started looking us over one by one. I remember her look as if it were yesterday. We were ready to eat lunch, so we ran into the house where Mom had prepared my favorite dish.

I loved tomatoes and rice. This was the meal of the day. I don't remember the rest of the meal. In later years, I developed an allergy to tomatoes. My older sister and I were given our food first because these people were going to take us away.

When the meal was over, my older sister and I were told to go with these two strangers. We had no idea we were being given away. It was only months later that we became resigned to the fact that we may never be going back home to our parents and siblings.

My dad apparently controlled my mom so completely until he was able to give away two of their children and get away with it. I don't know what he had told her, but she remained in the kitchen with the other siblings while we were being taken away.

There were no hugs, kisses, or goodbyes. We were just whisked away by these two strangers in their truck. Mom was a small-framed, four-feet-tall unassuming, quiet lady who wore her hair in two long thick braids. She went about her work singing and teaching us to sing. I never got to see her reaction to us being taken away.

When we got back together in later years, my older sister told me our dad had been abusive to our mom. When our foster parents took my sister back home, she was old enough to see and understand a lot of what took place. She and the other three siblings were given to our maternal uncle eventually.

It is documented that abusive partners control their mates to the degree of getting away with anything they want. Dad was no exception. He was able to pull off giving all of us away. He later said he wanted all of us to grow up in affluent homes and get an education. He said he knew he and my mom could never afford to do all of those things for us.

For years, I was at peace with that explanation. I later learned that abusive partners often get rid of their kids to hurt their mate. I am sure this hurt my mom very deeply. When families break, children hate to be separated from each other. They also do not like it when their parents separate.

When we were taken away, my sister was eight years old and I was six. My sister told me there had been a sibling between us that did not survive. She told me there were others that did not survive. Those lost siblings were spared the pain of this separation.

So here my sister and I sat, between these two strangers, not knowing where we were going or when we would return home to our parents and siblings. I remember having enough optimism or naïveté to think we must be going to something good. If I'd known the truth, perhaps I would have tried to run.

My older sister and I rode in silence. We were stunned. We had a head full of questions which we dared not ask these two big strangers. My older sister, who was always feisty and mouth almighty, somehow had surrendered her tongue to the cat. (This was an expression meaning a person couldn't talk due to fright.)

After a long ride, the couple parked the truck in front of a large house that had a very large yard. The lawn was green, and it appeared to have been manicured. The yard was fenced and had lots of flowers, shrubbery, flowering trees, orange trees, Japanese plum trees, mulberry trees, and cherry trees.

They helped us down out of the truck and led us into a beautifully decorated and spacious house. They took us on a tour of the house right away. We were not impressed. There was a large screened porch across the front for sitting. There was also a large screened back porch.

There were two bedrooms, and later, half of the back porch was converted into a bedroom. There was a nicely and colorfully decorated large bathroom with real indoor plumbing. The kitchen was large, and it had a large icebox. They purchased a refrigerator days later.

When the tour was over, my sister and I simultaneously burst into loud cries and tears. They took us to the store and bought ice cream and every good thing they thought would shut us up. That worked for a while. They called in the entire neighborhood of kids. That delighted us. We enjoyed that.

We all played until dark, at which time the other kids had to go home. We started crying again, but the big lady told us to shut up. We did. There was no contest. She gave us a bath in the big nice tub, had us to say our prayers, and then sent us to bed.

The lady woke us up to a delicious breakfast of grits, eggs, bacon, toast, orange juice, and milk. It seemed like the food and lodging were not so bad. Maybe this place was okay after all. The lady took us shopping for clothes, then to the nearby school and enrolled us the next day.

Things began to look better. There were more kids to play with. I loved learning, and we got to wear pretty new clothes and shoes every day. There was a lunchroom where we had good food every day. There was a playground with a merry-go-round, swings, a slide board, and lots of playmates.

The lady took us to church the next Sunday. When we got home, we had a scrumptious meal, and more neighborhood kids came to play. By now, things seemed so good until we did not think about home as much. We figured we would be going back someday. In the meantime, we would enjoy this place.

Children often serve as buffers for each other to help cushion hurt when they have to go through unpleasant situations. Sharing painful situations seems to make the situation better. Having other kids to play and talk with somehow eased the pain of being separated from our parents.

Soon we settled into a life of attending school through the week and playing with the neighborhood kids on weekends. Pretty soon, we were introduced to work. We were taught to wash dishes, sweep and mop the floor, dust the blinds and furniture, and rake the yard.

I was too short to reach the kitchen sink, so I was made to stand on an orange crate to wash the dishes. It seems this lady used every dish and pot in the kitchen to prepare meals. The pots were always sticky and hard to wash. It always took me a long time to wash the dishes.

No grease was allowed to be left on the dishes or pots. Everything had to be squeaky clean, or some form of punishment followed. We had to make our bed daily and keep our room clean. We were taught to wash our small clothing items on what was known then as a washboard.

Anything that was hung on the outdoor line had to be clean. There was no clothes dryer. We were taught to iron the clothes. Clothing was taken in from other families for laundering. Clothing had to look like they came from the dry cleaners when we were done with them.

The carefree life had ended, and now we were doing a lot of work. They owned a large orange grove across the street and lots of guava trees. We had access to the fruit at all times. Work was not unpleasant with all of the other good things about this place.

My sister and I still had to complete homework and study for school. There was very little playtime except early on Sunday afternoons after church services. Either the neighborhood kids came to see us, or we went to their houses. Adults always kept a close eye on us and reported any misbehavior.

The good things like going to school, playing with other kids, eating good food, wearing pretty clothes and shoes continued. We were given many children's books and nursery rhymes to read. We had bedtime storybooks and the Bible, from which our foster dad/uncle read to us.

The first Christmas, we were given toys, dolls, candies, nuts, and more pretty clothes. The lady's aunt also gave us toys and clothing items, which she brought over to be placed under the Christmas tree. Pleasant things can distract kids for a long time. We were no exception.

My sister and I were distracted from the idea of returning home. We went on with the business of living and adjusting as best we could for displaced kids. We had adjusted to a point of everything seemingly going fine. It seemed as if we were going to be here forever, so we may as well adjust to it.

As I look back over the years, it seems as though we sold out our parental affection for the life of luxury we were enjoying. Or could it have been our way of coping with a situation over which neither of us had any control? Children tend to have amazing abilities to adapt to adverse situations.

Left Alone

I thought things were going pretty well for my sister and me. As we got older, my sister rebelled and started disrespecting our foster parents. One Sunday morning before church, she broke a bottle of catsup. Our foster mom had gone to visit her sister who lived nearby for a few minutes.

I was on the front porch when she returned. I heard a terrible ruckus in the kitchen. She was shouting and saying threatening things to my sister. I went into the kitchen, where she apparently had caught my sister with some evidence of the event. We were both punished.

Things began to take a downhill turn as my sister began to rebel more and more. Whenever she did some type of mischief, we both got whipped because she would not admit to what she had done. There were times I was whipped without ever knowing why. You didn't question the judgment of elders.

A lot of parents punished in that manner during those days. If the perpetrator lied, everybody got whipped. If the adult said you did it, whether you did or not, you got punished. My sister gave the lady a lot of sass, so the lady took her back home to our parents. I was left alone with these strangers.

By the time my sister was taken back, our dad had given all of my siblings away. He gave four of them to our biological uncle. He had my mom committed to a rest home for no reason. Mom was devastated, but she never protested as far as we know.

Mom had apparently been traumatized by years of abuse and having her children taken away. She was forced to live among psychiatric patients for several years. The staff and social workers who worked with her discovered she was not a mental case. She was transferred to an intermediate care facility.

When I became a married adult, I inquired about taking Mom home to live with me. For some reason, one doctor would not allow us to take her home. He said when a patient had been in an environment for a long time, it was not good to move them. We accepted his answer, and there she remained until she died at age ninety-two.

My foster mom (who was alleged to be my aunt) became what I perceived as abusive to me as far as beatings went. The abuses occurred between good times. Church life and school life made existence bearable and pleasant. My music and associations with friends also made life bearable.

The good meals, the new clothes and shoes, and all the other good things continued between the cyclic beatings. I was allowed to belong to the Girl Scouts of America, the school band, the church choir, and even to attend summer camps.

Another thing in my favor was that I got along well with my teachers and other schoolmates. I met a friend who has indeed been a friend through the years. I met L. Townsend in the fourth grade. We hit it off really well. We both loved to laugh, and we enjoyed the same activities.

LT had a good mom and dad and a normal life. She lived in the suburbs of town, but I was allowed to visit her sometimes. Her mom, dad, and siblings were very kind and sweet. Knowing L. and her family somehow cushioned me from the abuses. LT and I are still friends today.

Our lives have paralleled each other from fourth grade until now. Even though we were in different parts of the world, we got married the same time. We had similar careers and retired within one year of each other. I could discuss anything with LT, and I believe she feels the same way about me. She still remembers me on my birthday and holidays.

Another buffer to the abuses was my foster dad. (He was supposedly also my uncle.) He was what a lot of people called henpecked. He was not henpecked as far as I was concerned: he was just a gentle giant. He showed sympathy for me many times during the severe punishments.

One evening, dinner was withheld from me for some trivial reason. When mother dear left to go to church, my foster dad gave me money and told me to go to the community grocery store and buy myself something to eat. I purchased some food and made a meal.

It was traditional for a lot of moms in those days to have their children call them "Mother dear" in an attempt to be proper. It was supposed to lend an air of sophistication. With kids, Mother dear came out as "Mud-dear."

On another occasion, I was fearful of asking MD for money to buy a Christmas gift. We drew names at school, and of all the names in the school, I drew LT.'s name. Because I was afraid to ask for gift money, I waited until the last minute to ask. MD refused to give me any money so I headed off to school embarrassed and empty-handed.

On his way to work early that morning, my faithful foster dad had left me some money atop one of the shrubs beside the front gate. The paper bills were wet from the morning dew. I was able to buy a box of chocolate-covered cherries for LT from the corner grocery store. That was all I could afford.

LT admired and loved the chocolate-covered cherries. She still eats them today. She was eating some when I visited her for Christmas last year. Fortunately the candy box itself had a Christmas design in those days, so I did not need to buy wrapping paper.

Incidents were less stressful when my foster dad or aunt intervened. They had a way of helping me behind Mother dear's back or manipulating the situation to make her think she had done a good thing. MD was a people pleaser. She was always trying to please a friend of hers at church.

Her friend had a daughter who was a little older than I was. MD imitated and copied everything her friend did for her daughter. She was determined to keep me in vogue with her friend's daughter, which was a good thing for me.

MD had no children of her own. This friend was her role model as to what a mom should be like. She wanted to please her friend with whatever she did for me. This was her friend's only child. Her friend was from a large family, and most of her own family members had children.

All of the children in this friend's family as well her own daughter wore nice clothes, took piano lessons, were in the school band, the local Girl Scout troop, and participated in all church functions for young people. I was given many advantages because of this competition between our parents.

Parents whom I talked with during my life and nursing career told me they were not automatic parents, although they were once kids themselves. They had to learn how to be parents. Others have totally missed the parenting thing. This is why mentoring by teachers and other significant adults is so important for kids.

The good things I experienced served to shape my outlook on life. The Girl Scout meetings allowed me to learn to do arts and crafts and other age-appropriate activities with my fellow scouts. The scout leader was a mothering type of woman who gave us weekly positive experiences.

The nightly summer campfires of singing and roasting marshmallows were fun. I had the opportunity to learn how to get along with people. I even pleased MD because my dishwashing skills became quicker and neater. I became a better housekeeper.

Mother dear was pleased that I also had a new resolve to keep my closet neat, which I did. When it was time to sell Girl Scout cookies, she advertised the sales among her church people. My self-esteem soared over my accomplishments. I still feel the pride of having participated in the local Girl Scout troop.

Other good things happened. The lady with whom my Mother dear was in competition had given her daughter piano lessons for many years. Our choir director was young and wanted to see more children learn to play the piano. MD jumped at the opportunity and allowed me to take music lessons.

This was a blessing in disguise and something I wanted very much. I never thought music lessons would happen because MD held money tightly. I thought someone would have to be giving free lessons if she were going to pay for them. The lessons at the church cost $3.00 per hour.

MD's friend and competitor's daughter placed me on programs to sing at every church function. This allowed me to grow up singing in church. The daughter of mother dear's competition enjoyed playing and showing off her skills. Having me sing gave her a chance for unlimited playing.

This friend's sister was over the majorettes in the band. She also belonged to our church. She talked with MD, and I was allowed to be a majorette. Being a majorette in the band required that we learn to play an instrument. I learned to play the trumpet.

Pretty soon, I was playing hymns on the piano in churches and earning money to play around town. I even sang at a school competition and wowed my schoolmates, who did not know I sang. Children need to have their self-esteems boosted, especially misplaced kids. Activities allow this.

As I look back over my childhood days, on a scale from one to ten, I would say they were a ten, excluding the awful beatings. With the situations I have faced in life, in retrospect, I appreciate the beatings. They perhaps kept me out of a lot of mischief that I would have gotten into.

Parents had a way of putting the fear of God into their children. None of my schoolmates ever went to jail or prison. We all got beaten or punished for misdeeds. One of my MD's tenant's sons started stealing at an early age. MD owned and rented out several apartments on our property. This mom got on top of the problem and nipped it in the bud.

This son was around eight or nine years old when he went in the teacher's purse and stole money. When the crime was discovered, his mom was summoned to the school. She beat the poor child unmercifully in front of everyone.

He tried one more act of thievery from the corner grocery store. In those days, people did not call the police. His mom found out, made it good with the storekeeper, and just about killed her son again. He grew into a fine, upstanding young man who pursued a military career.

The harsh discipline channeled that young man and me in the right direction at an early age. I believe this was part of the footstep-ordering process that governed my life. In those days, telephones were not in most homes. Somehow news always quickly got to our parents if we acted out in the community.

Teachers and other adults were allowed to freely discipline other people's children. Children had a respect for adults that is not seen in today's American society. The degree of beatings we got could have easily been classified as abuse in today's world.

Sadly, some parents and adults do go overboard with harsh discipline and end up in the courts. Adults sometimes discipline children while they are very angry and enter into the realm of abuse. Unfortunately, my MD had a temper, and I felt the wrath of it with each flogging.

In her attempt to see that I grew up to be a proper adult, MD always tried to expose me to the right people and events. There was one really bad street in town where crime flourished. There were all sorts of criminal-minded people afoot on that street all the time. I was strongly warned never to go there. I drove through that street as an adult.

Parents also chose our playmates. If a child had a name for being "bad," we were not allowed to play with them. We were to avoid being around girls who hung out with boys. A schoolmate in a higher grade became with child. We were forbidden to have anything to do with her.

Wrong peer associations can definitely bring out the worst in some children. This is why parents forbade us to play with certain children while we were growing up. The new babysitter affectionately known as the television exposes children to all kinds of undesirable as well as good knowledge.

In the absence of learning and exposure, the television has filled in the knowledge gap for many people. When God is ordering our footsteps, we can step off the path in our own self-will and rebel. We have the option to choose the right or the wrong path.

Even though God will order our steps, he gives us free will as human beings. Adam and Eve, our first parents, were given free will. They were warned not to eat of the fruit of the tree of the knowledge of good and evil. Adam was told what would happen if they did. Read Genesis 2:9, 16, 17.

God did not stand over them and force them not to eat of the forbidden fruit. Instead, he allowed them the freedom to live in the same garden as the tree. He did not lock the tree away or remove it from the garden in which they resided. Exercising free will is what gets most of us in trouble.

When we have the choice to stop or run a red light, we may exercise our will to run the light. We have been warned what could happen, and it is the law to stop at the light. Whatever happens to us is not always God's will, so we bring things on our own selves when we exercise free will.

In many instances of this writing, you will see where I chose to exercise free will rather than to patiently allow God to order my steps. My parents wanted me to remain with them and allow them to send me to College. They had plans for me that I did not know about.

I chose to take matters into my own hands and ran away from two different situations. Things turned out okay in the end, but how much better they may have been had I done things in order? We are usually obsessed with the idea of taking the path of least resistance or the most comfortable route.

Years after looking back over the running away incidents, I can warn kids about running away. I have been able to counsel people who were contemplating running away from situations. Others who were contemplating suicide have been counseled to embrace life. All of them are still alive.

Even when we miss God, he is able to order our footsteps in a way so as to help someone else. We may not have gone the route we planned or someone planned for us, but we did get to a destination that resulted in some good happening.

"The steps of a good man are ordered by the Lord: and he delighteth in his way" Psalm 37:23. "Thy word is a lamp unto my feet, and a light unto my path" Psalm 119:105. We should pray to the Lord to order our steps in all things.

Nursing, my earliest heart's desire

As far as my recollection serves me, being a nurse was an early desire in my life. Being raised as an only child away from my siblings allowed me to observe other people's lives. Whenever I saw suffering, I wanted to remedy it. My life was pretty much regimented like a soldier.

After growing up and talking with my siblings, they told me they had not grown up with the stability and structure I had in my life. They did have adults and teachers who mentored them from time to time. Two sisters did not complete high school until later years. Each learned a trade and was able to carve out a good life.

After learning of the siblings' plight, I began to appreciate the discipline and having a consistent life. The corporal punishment was a bit much; however, it instilled within me the knowledge that all of life's actions have consequences.

I learned that the discipline would come in handy for studying and working toward a goal. When discipline has been instilled in children, they have what they need to accomplish purposes in life.

Children need consistency in their lives. Part of the consistency in my life was getting to school and church services on time. I had times allotted for study and for every area of my life. I received a small allowance for jobs well done.

Home chores had to be completed after school assignments were completed. There was no Saturday-morning sleeping in. Most adults of that generation instilled in children a sense of responsibility and work ethics. They had a no-nonsense approach to child rearing.

Fun was derived from playing with the neighborhood children, attending church activities, and from the school's extracurricular fellowships with other students. The harsh beatings continued from time to time mainly, I believe, on general principle.

Elementary and high school were good years. I made the honor roll much of the time. I was also considered the best reader in the past in our elementary school class. The schoolteachers discovered during elementary school that I had art abilities, which they put to good use.

During the elementary school years, our teachers tried to expose us to much of what life had to offer along with schoolwork. Periodically they would bring in a magician, a hypnotist, bank personnel, and even Santa Claus to teach us some lessons and to amuse us.

I established a lot of friendships, some of which are still in my life today. We telephone each other and chat from time to time. I was taught a lot from the assortment of people our teachers brought into the school to teach and/or amuse us.

Several magicians came from time to time. Kids seemed to enjoy them more than the other performers. We all enjoyed seeing a rabbit pulled from a hat, a woman sawed in half, the coin trick, and other feats. One day, a different magician came. We were required to form a line and ask him questions about our future one by one.

This particular magician had a light bulb in his hand. Somehow the bulb would light up when we asked him our particular question. There was no visible power source to the bulb. That trick in itself was amazing to us. The bulb lit up for "yes" answers and went out for "no" answers.

My question was, "Will I be a nurse when I grow up? The bulb's light went out. The magician also shook his head in the negative, and then he said, "No, you will not become a nurse." I soon forgot about him until I had completed nurses' training.

I could have stored that information in my mind's computer and never pursued a nursing career. Had it not been for my forgetting the magician's answer all those years, I might have never been a nurse. I could have agreed with him and never reached my goal.

"Death and life are in the power of the tongue" Proverbs 18:21. We have what we continue to say with our mouths. If we always say, "Things are bad in my life," things will remain that way. Continue to say, "I'll never succeed," and you will not succeed.

This brings up another point. While there are a lot of true prophets in the earth, we do have to be aware that there are also false prophets. There are God-sent prophets, and there are people who inherited the gift of seeing into the future. Some of these have never yielded their gifts for God's use.

There are other seers who went to school to learn how to read fortunes. I was offered the opportunity to do so. Being a God-fearing person, I chose not to play with his gifts. Many secrets can be revealed from God when we totally yield ourselves to him through studying his word, prayer, and fasting.

In the second chapter of Daniel in the King James Version of the Bible, the king had a vision which no magician, soothsayer, seer, or Chaldean could interpret. The king sent out a decree to slay all of them because they could not interpret his dream nor could they tell him what he had dreamed.

When Daniel learned of the king's hasty death decree, he requested permission of the king to give him time to seek his God for the answer. After Daniel and his companions went before their God and prayed, Daniel was given the dream and its interpretation in a night vision.

Daniel told the king what he had dreamed and the interpretation. Daniel later told the king, "But there is a God in heaven that revealeth secrets, and maketh known to the king Nebuchadnezzar what shall be in the latter days" Daniel 2:28.

A goal thwarter almost derailed my College plans. College should have been my first priority. Instead, I chose to get married. That would have been fine, except I entered into marriage with College in the back of my head. Future College plans were never discussed mutually with my future spouse.

To anyone planning a College career and marriage, both parties need to be in agreement with the College plan. Otherwise, it can be a point of contention that eats at the fiber of the marriage. Marriage is an endeavor that requires the cooperation of both parties.

After a few months of having to come home and prepare meals, do laundry, study, play for the church, function as a minister's wife and work, I was ready to chuck all of it. I longed for the carefree single life again. It took a lot of fortitude and determination to complete College.

At the end of one of the semesters, I had all of my credits except three. In order to graduate in sequence, I needed to go to another College during the summer and get the three credits in psychology. The nearest College was the University of Miami.

Arrangements were made, and I enrolled for the required six-week course. All of those students who were my age really made me regret not completing College before marriage. My roommate was always out somewhere having fun after classes. I felt obligated to stay in the dorm or the library since I was not single.

Finally, the six weeks were over. I returned to the University of Florida, where I was able to graduate on schedule. Another goal thwarter cropped up during the weeks prior to graduation for my bachelor's degree. This thwarter was the most difficult for me.

Three scholarship offers presented themselves again. Dr. DW, our pediatrics professor, offered me the opportunity to obtain my master's degree in pediatrics. Dr. JS offered me the opportunity to earn my master's in psychiatric nursing, and Dr. VP offered the opportunity for masters in public health.

Here was a grand opportunity to earn a master's degree and not have to pay for it. I loved all three areas. I quickly thought of taking public health; that way, it would allow me to work with children and all other disciplines of nursing.

As I rushed home with the news, it never occurred to me this goal would be thwarted. I was told, "You have been gone a lot already. When are you going to stay home and be a wife?" There went my aspirations for a master's degree. I earned a master's in theology several years later.

My early lesson learned from childhood is that all actions have consequences. Choosing marriage over education had its consequences. We must make choices during our entire lifetime. Right or wrong choices often determine our destiny.

"Without counsel purposes are disappointed, but in the multitude of counselors they are established" Proverbs 15:22. We may have counsel and not heed it. As we look back over what our parents, teachers, ministers, and elders taught us, we can glean much counsel. Are we following it?

When parents disagree with a marriage choice, they see something in the mate that will possibly cause problems sooner or later within the marriage. Since they spend many years molding them, good parents want what is best for their children.

Despite the things that had happened in my rearing as a child, the parents I knew still wanted to ensure my future success. When I mentioned marriage to them, they verbally expressed their disapproval of my timing and my choice. They had dreams of me graduating from College before marriage.

They disagreed with my choice of mate because he had not completed high school and he was going to take me into his mom's house to live. He would have to work a few years in order for us to afford our own place to live. To my parents, this was a poor excuse of a husband.

My spouse and I worked between my schooling, and we purchased a nice brand-new home. I continued my education, but the hours away from home eventually took their toll. My spouse took adult education classes to complete high school.

It seemed we had proved my parents wrong. But the struggles could have been avoided had I listened to their counsel. People often say, "Opposites attract," but being unequally yoked has its downside. When couples have common interests more serenity seems to prevail.

"Be ye not unequally yoked together with unbelievers: for what fellowship hath righteousness with unrighteousness? And what communion hath light with darkness?" 2 Corinthians 6:14 This scripture refers to Christians joining forces with sinners, but can apply to any situation, especially marriage.

Paul the Apostle knew that if those who were Christian fellowshipped with those who were not, there would be problems. When a Christian goes into the bar, sits and drinks even a Coke with a non-Christian, pretty soon his ability to lead someone to Christ is disabled.

Those who look upon the situation, both believers and nonbelievers will often say, "I knew there was nothing to him all along." "He is just a hypocrite." "Let not then your good be evil spoken of" Romans 14:16. Unfortunately, no one sees his behavior as that of a friend.

They are unequally yoked in the eyes of all, and no amount of explaining justifies what is seen. When parents warn children of a prospective mate, at least listen to what they are telling you, and weigh your decision.

One morning prior to leaving for the thirty-five-mile commute to classes, I mentioned to my spouse that I had a sore throat and a cold. In his quest to assist me to wellness quickly, he made a hot toddy for me to drink. Being a teetotaler, I had never drunk alcohol in my life.

He quickly made the toddy while I completed getting dressed and gathering up my books to leave. As I was leaving out of the door, he said, "Drink this." Happy to get any relief, I gulped it down quickly. I had hardly swallowed the mixture before I began feeling woozy.

I thought to myself, *I guess I had better lie down so these effects can wear off. I don't want to drive feeling this way.* As I lay down, sleep fell upon me immediately. I slept all day, all night, and awoke the next morning feeling fine. The sore throat was gone.

I never woke up once to eat, drink, or go to the rest room. I asked my spouse what was in the drink. He replied, "Honey, lemon juice and gin." I never touched any alcohol since that time. Anything that could render me that helpless was best left alone.

Besides, I was the laughingstock of the class and the instructor when I told them what happened. My prior attendance record was perfect until that fateful day. I could have decided I liked that drink and ended up being an alcoholic.

Most of the people I knew at that time admired my tenacity to return to College, commute, and go through all I was going through to complete College. There were others who stood back and criticized, saying, "All of that education will make you crazy." "College is for kids."

Many people allow the embarrassment of age, opinions of others and other factors to hinder them from pursuing their most desired goals. Some have been heard to say, "My kids have all finished school, and I am ashamed to go back." "I am scared I won't make good grades."

Alibis and excuses sound really good only to the ones who are making them. Think about what you will be doing five years down the road if you do take that step and go to school. Think again about what you will be doing if you don't take that step and go.

Sure, it takes money to do things. Some Colleges still have scholarships and loan programs. Try and stash a little cash from that job with College in mind. Most of us waste a lot of money on frivolous things that are thrown away a few years later. Basically most of us get and do what we want to do.

I have seen entire households of furniture and clothing thrown on roadside trash piles. Money was spent to purchase those items by someone at one time in their lives. Now the merchandise is useless and unwanted. Those items were considered as very valuable at one time in their lives. Start planning today.

How many times have you said, "One day I am going to go and see about enrolling in nurses' training" or some other career of your dreams? Procrastination and laziness cause many people to leave this earth without ever putting a finger toward a desired goal.

There are other times when we have aspirations and certain things occur in our lives to spur us on to our goals. Although I had the inner desire to go on to College after high school, circumstances allowed me to procrastinate. My marriage was just getting started, and I found myself busy with almost no time for nurses' training.

My working at the downtown dry goods store was panning out well. I was learning to decorate the store windows, check stock, and to master a number of job-related skills. The income was fairly good for a high school graduate. My coworkers were pleasant to work with and life was good.

About a year into the work, I hit a snag. Cleaning the rest rooms was a part of my job, and until now I had no problem with it. This day, someone had really messed up the ladies' room's commode, floor, and walls with body waste.

Cleaning the rest room was now a problem. It seems everyone in the building started paging and calling my name to come and clean the rest room. I had already cleaned the rest rooms the night before, so I could not imagine why the calls were so urgent.

Whether this was a malicious prank or a really sick person who visited the rest room remains a mystery to me today. Being the youngest employee and basically the new kid on the block put me in the position to have to clean the rest rooms. My trainer/mentor was off that day.

My first impulse when I beheld the mess was to grab my purse, run, and never look back. The couple who sat on the porch that fateful Sunday waiting to take me and my sister with them had taught me to stick with a job. They had taught me to do the best job I can do no matter how unpleasant.

As a surgeon would do, I donned gloves and an apron and covered my face with a paper mask. After all, this was a serious job. I cleaned the rest room from top to bottom with the strongest detergents I could find in the broom closet. I sprayed the place with deodorizer.

When I got home that evening, I practically scrubbed the skin off my body to get rid of the stench and the dirty feeling. I pondered what could have happened to propel another human being to do such a thing and to walk away with no apology or explanation. Surely they must have felt ashamed.

My foster parents had lived through hard times, and their opinion and teachings were that you do not walk away from a job. A new level of respect came to me from the job following that incident. Everyone commented on how well the job was done and how much better the whole place smelled.

It seems some employees thought I would surely leave or create a scene. When that didn't happen, everyone began to be nicer to me. I found myself in line for better things on the job, but by then I had decided it was time to move on. That incident was the spur in my saddle that caused me to move on.

During that period of time, I received a nice-sized income tax refund. The refund helped me to pivot on to cosmetology school. I took a day off, drove the several miles away to the town where the school was located, and enrolled for the next term.

I gave a proper notice to the job and moved on. I found out real early that when we do not take advantage of the opportunities to learn and further ourselves, we are doomed to practice whatever menial chores life hands out. After completing cosmetology, I pursued my nursing career.

I worked cosmetology at a friend's shop off and on between everything else. My dream of being a nurse never died. Kismet, destiny, fate, or the hand of God (I choose to believe it was the hand of God), caused the cosmetology school to relocate in the same building as the nursing school.

This move put the nursing school in my path and allowed me to complete the associate's degree training in nursing. The hand of God always seemed to be there to lead me on to the next level, especially when I was willing to move.

My journey through College was fraught with times of delays, procrastination, some laziness, but I intended to finish someday. Someday is the big time we all look forward to. Someday may never come, so do what you can now to accomplish your goals.

Had I known such a beautiful career awaited me, perhaps I would have gone straight through College and Bible College. It seemed I was always climbing to a higher goal. The ultimate dream and goal were always in my mind. I had no intention of letting go until I had accomplished all of them.

My brother and I were recently discussing how each of us reached certain goals. With each of us there were mentors that God seemed to purposely put in our paths who pushed us further. He was pushed with his music while I was pushed with my nurses' training.

Many of our teachers and people around us saw in each of us a resolve to accomplish our goals, and many of them seemingly stepped out of the shadows to help us. When you are surrounded with wise people, they behold your efforts and will often do what they can to further you along.

My brother and I shared the same singing instructions from our dad. We both, along with our other siblings, were sung to by our mom. Before we were all given away, these same parents taught us the Lord's Prayer, certain scriptures, and common manners.

NURSING GOALS
ACCOMPLISHED

Each nursing school's graduation came and was celebrated. Upon graduation from the two-year school, our professors warned us that the entry level for nursing practice would quickly become the baccalaureate degree. With this information, I decided to work a while and then return to College. The doctoral level promises to be the future entry level.

The local hospital gladly received me because I had trained there and they knew I had also been employed under a top community surgeon in the past. The salary was better than any I had ever earned. I was tempted to settle in and forget about going on for the bachelor's degree.

After working a couple of years, I decided to pursue the next level of nursing at the nearest College. The College happened to be approximately thirty-five miles away. I took a day off from work, drove to the College, and enrolled for classes. Before long, I was attending classes.

After trying to commute and struggle with studies, my spouse and I decided it would be better for me to live in the dormitory at least until I could get adjusted to College life. The studies were very heavy, and I found myself staying up all night to do reports and study.

Eventually I adjusted to the heavy studying and library work. Those first weeks were a sort of boot camp. I met a young lady from a deep Southern state. She told me she was from the South and was somewhat of a rebel. We studied together and got reports together. She ceased her rebelling.

With our concerted effort, we made good grades. We graduated and went our separate ways. We neglected getting mutual addresses and phone numbers. We both just faded into the woodwork, never to hear from each other again. I even forgot her last name.

Race relations were not the best during those years. Less than 1 percent of the thirty thousand student population at my College was Afro Americans. Some of the younger students were very militant and spitting venom. They wanted to pull me into boycotts and other incendiary activities, which I avoided.

I was married and commuting, struggling to maintain a B average, and spending government money to go to school. I had gone through so much already. Nothing was going to deter my route to my target of completing College. I felt like with a College degree I would be in a better bargaining position.

Some of the same students flunked out and went home. They were never heard from again. This was one of those times I had to consider consequences. It was now or never with my education. Without a degree, I may have had to return to cleaning the toilets involuntarily.

The years prior to attending nursing school had found me singing in the mass meetings, marching and participating in the rights movements. This had been one of the means by which I had access to nursing education. Both Colleges I attended had just started opening their doors and reaching out to minorities.

One night, an announcement came into one of the mass meetings where I was attending. The local nursing College was recruiting minorities. I immediately signed up and was accepted. Later in my education, the four-year College where these students wanted to start a revolution had also just started granting access to each of us.

To join the revolutionists would have derailed and thwarted my educational goals. There is a time to participate in just causes, and this was not the time for me. We cannot allow our emotions to always dictate our actions. Prayer and careful thought work better.

Florence Nightingale, our leader, left some examples for making strides not only in nursing, but in all areas of life. She cooperated with the political system to bring about changes. A vote in the right place at the right time for the right person speaks volumes and does much.

The desire to become a nurse had been a goal branded in my spirit since childhood. Sometimes, when goals are placed on hold, they can never be restarted. I was passionate about reaching my goal, so I weighed my actions at that time. I could not afford to forfeit this goal.

Staying in school finally reaped its rewards. Not only was I offered scholarships to go further in nurses' training, but I was also offered several high-paying jobs. My College's doctorate law program also offered me a chance to pursue a degree in legal studies.

Doors started opening everywhere as a result of me sticking with my educational goals. The sheepskin (diploma) appeared to be such an insignificant-looking piece of paper, but it carried much weight. Through it, the Lord opened many doors for me.

Attending Bible College had also been a longtime goal of mine. I had been taught scriptures for so long and had read the Bible from cover to cover more than one time. Out of all of the reading, there was much I still did not understand. I needed someone to explain its meaning to me.

Gaining an understanding of the word was my only reason for wanting to go to Bible College. When I started attending Bible school, the school's founder informed all of us that we needed to study the Bible and obtain degrees along with keeping the anointing in our lives.

"All Spirit and no Word equals fanaticism. All Word and no Spirit equals formalism," according to our pastor. The professor at the Bible College warned us that a time will come when those carrying God's Word will need educational credentials. We also need to be balanced.

With my nurses' training behind me, I began to feel appreciation for the couple who was sitting on the front porch of my biological parents' home a few years ago. These were the people who laid the foundation in me for getting an education. In their special way, they parented me.

How often do we fail to appreciate people before it is too late? Not only did they prepare me to get an education, they instilled principles in me that have helped to guide me through the years. For someone who had no child-rearing experience, they instilled some worthwhile qualities in me.

Godly parental guidance and protection from the deleterious elements in our town and environment were provided for me. I was allowed to participate in wholesome organizations and activities. Every advantage for educational advancement was given to me.

As children, we did not see the good things our biological or foster parents were trying to provide for us. The lady who took us in had a need to mother. We needed mothering. She did her best to send us on our life's journey fairly well equipped.

Our teachers were also very instrumental in mentoring and encouraging all of us to get a sound education. We were told of the benefits of getting at least a high school education. Every child was given the opportunity to excel. Many of us were given scholarships.

Some students made average grades all through school. I was amazed to learn years later that some of those students completed College and/or trades and were doing well at teaching or some other profitable high-profile jobs. Another student who basically made a lot of C and D grades went on to be a movie stuntman in Hollywood.

Three special needs students were mainstreamed before mainstreaming was ever heard about. They were allowed to be socially promoted despite their mental challenges. They were made to feel as though they were just as good as anyone else. They marched with everyone else at graduation time. All through school, they were mentored like everyone else.

Two of the special needs students passed away at an early age. The third one is still living and is being cared for by his family. Special needs children and adults are not always accorded the dignity they should have. Only recently has society attempted to include special needs people in the flow of life.

These parents taught me how to respect and get along with people. They taught me to respect differences in people and never to hate anyone. They taught me the futility of jealousy. "For love is strong as death; jealousy is cruel as the grave: the coals thereof are coals of fire, which hath a most vehement flame" Song of Solomon 8:6.

Bible College

By now, I had completed my nursing education, gone through marital dissolution, worked for several years, moved away and purchased a home, traveled internationally, worked in South Florida, and then resumed my Bible College studies. After several single years, I entered into an abusive matrimonial relationship.

By the time I reached my master's level, the Bible College had developed a domestic violence institute. The entire curriculum was devoted to comprehensive courses about domestic violence. Domestic violence courses became prerequisites for graduation.

At least two of my female professors had survived abusive marriages. They were well versed on the subject and presented the most current and relevant information about domestic violence. They wanted students to be well-informed about abuse.

It was no coincidence that the institute existed during my time as a student. I was able to see my life of abuse very clearly in the content of the courses. I lived in denial for several years, but the courses forced me to face my issues.

We learned that domestic violence affects 90 to 95 percent of female victims and about 5 percent of males. Annually, six million women are battered by their partners. DV affects all classes of society, regardless of race or status in life.

Intimate partners commit 50 percent of murders perpetrated on women. The most common cause of serious injury to women is due to domestic violence. Many cases of domestic violence go unreported. Women tend to protect their abusers. I was no exception.

I attended a recent seminar on DV that was presented locally. One surprising fact that came out of the seminar and hit close to home was that perpetrators often choke their victims to death. My partner had attempted to choke me early in marriage. In the past, choking left no visible wounds, and the perpetrators got away with the crime.

Had I not spoken out loudly and forcefully when the perpetrator started after my neck, I might have been a statistic today. Seeing those hands coming at my throat triggered a response in me that came out of me quickly, spontaneously, and verbally forceful. The perpetrator backed down. From that point on, abuse was verbal.

This is usually the sequence of domestic violence. The perpetrator starts testing to see what the victim will endure. Every episode that is tolerated or allowed leads to bigger and more frequent episodes. I was experiencing the testing stage.

Women often leave repeatedly, only to return to a deteriorating relationship. They think their leaving will shock the perpetrator into doing better. This only threatens his sense of loss of power and control and puts the victim in greater danger.

Bible College continued

Prior to getting married, I had enjoyed attending Bible College and life was flowing along nicely. It seemed as though nothing could go wrong. I had acquired a lot of friends at the Bible College, and I continued to travel during breaks. My life's activities consisted of working, singing, and playing music.

A friend invited me to come to a Saturday night prayer meeting in a private home. I visited the prayer meeting, and many of the people there knew me. The lady in charge had been informed that I played music. She asked me to sing and play the keyboard for their weekly prayer meetings.

Since I was rarely busy on Saturday nights, I accepted the engagement. Traveling within the state was one requirement of the job. We traveled and held services. Videos were made of each service, and we watched them on Sunday afternoons.

One lady started trying to matchmake and introduced me to her pastor. His wife of almost fifty years had passed away. After hearing my tapes, the minister and his sister started attending the prayer meetings regularly. He purchased some of my tapes. The matchmaker said he listened to them all the time.

What I did not know and the man did not know is that the lady doing the matchmaking was leading him to believe I was interested in him and leading me to believe he was interested in me. She kept encouraging me to go out with him.

For months, I avoided going out with him. I did not want to date a preacher. He continued to ask me out. By then, most of the ladies thought I was giving up a good catch. People who knew him kept encouraging me to at least give the fellow a break. Everyone seemed to think we were perfect for each other.

Some ladies were telling me, "He's a preacher, and he's a good man." I continued to run and avoid the relationship. I did not want to be a preacher's wife a second time. The preacher's wife's role is unique and demanding, but it has its rewards. I felt like I could gain rewards some other way.

Whatever problems the minister faces, his wife faces, especially if she is aware of the problems. The position is perfect for impacting people's lives for the kingdom of God. If they both love the Lord and are guided by his Holy Spirit, lives are changed positively forever.

If domestic violence is involved, the congregation gets a skewed view of their leaders. They may see the pastor as a knight in shining armor and never see what his family is actually going through. I tried to adjust for the sake of the people, but I could not be a hypocrite and a pretender.

Many minister's wives remain in domestic violence relationships because they consider what it would do to the people if they left the relationship. While this is a noble cause, it is not a good reason to continually endure domestic violence. Leaders who are in such a case need to come clean.

Bible College
and elopement

Prior to eloping, I had several days off work. I had planned to spend time with my family in South Florida. I mentioned this to the minister. Quickly he asked if he could go with me. I informed him that he would have to get separate lodging since we were not married. I had no idea he was serious about going.

Upon his insistence, we went in his automobile. He insisted it was larger and more comfortable. As we traveled and talked, we found we had a lot in common. We both loved music, travel, church work, and we knew some of the same people.

Everyone had said he was such a good person until I felt safe with him. We began conversing on our way down South. The conversation was innocent and fairly innocuous. We never discussed love or affection. We kept the conversation on the surface. and Platonic.

After a long period of silence, a quick proposal of marriage to me by him followed. I told him I didn't really know him and he didn't know me. He stated if I would trust him, he would trust me. I said yes, thinking I would have time to weasel out of this one. I had no idea that he was really serious and that this marriage could occur all in one day.

The minister knew about these things, so he solicited the help of one of my family members to pull the marriage together. A preacher was obtained from one of the churches I had played for in the area. A family friend worked for the courthouse, and a license was obtained very quickly. I kept thinking, *surely this will not happen today.*

How wrong I was. By noontime, everything was arranged. The wife of the preacher who performed the ceremony ran a day care at the church. Part of the staff and my family comprised the audience. Everything was falling in place like clockwork, and things were happening too fast for me.

I had neglected to pray that morning and the night before because this trip was consuming so much of my time. I had not taken time to hear the Holy Spirit about any of these events. This was a perfect example of irresponsibly going into marriage lightly and unadvisedly.

Elopement is a very dangerous venture, especially if you have not known each other as longtime friends. A mate who insists on a quickie marriage has something to hide. He/she wants to entrap you before you find out the truth and sort out the facts. Love will wait.

After the marriage, we went to a nearby motel to spend the night. Immediately I felt like I had made a grave mistake. We had not thought this thing out, and we really did not know each other. He seemed quite comfortable with me, but all of a sudden I wanted to undo everything.

I had taken another oath to love, cherish, obey, etc., until death do us part. I had suddenly locked myself into a situation that I had to live with and make it work. There was no romance or love, and everything seemed so surreal. As time went by, I also began to feel embarrassed because I had done a stupid thing.

The next day, we drove the 325 miles back home. We got dressed and went to his church. People began to gather, and I was introduced as the pastor's new wife. Most of the people respected the pastor's decision to choose a wife. They treated me with respect. The first sister to arrive sang with me as I tried out the organ before services began. We sang together like we had always known each other.

Everyone was just as surprised about the marriage as I was. We later had a formal ceremony with a reception and all the works. Family, friends, well-wishers, coworkers, church people, classmates and instructors from the Bible College and prayer groups all attended and wished us well.

I soon began to feel like things were going to be okay. I returned to work. We lived at my condominium at first, and then we moved to his spacious home. The house appeared as though no one had lived there for a long time, and much repair work needed to be done. Cobwebs were everywhere.

We moved in before the repairs were done. I questioned something that I did not understand, and a second incident of abuse occurred. The preacher became angry and reached for my throat to choke me. Earlier, during our stay at my place, he had initiated an unprovoked angry verbal confrontation.

The verbal abuse continued on many occasions. I was told by him to "Get out!" of his house on several occasions for no reason. He would later come and find me at my residence and ask me to come back home. Dutifully, I would return home. One time, a prophet told me God wanted me to go back home to my husband. I went back.

We went on a cruise, and he shoved me. I almost fell down a flight of stairs. I was not aware that all of this was abusive behavior. One of my work supervisors recognized my plight and told me I was an abused woman. I vehemently disputed her and lived in denial for a long time.

She gave me leave time to go for counseling sessions. The counselors told me I had to bring my husband in order to help us both. He refused, stating that the church should handle such things. The perpetrator would have been the counselor for the help sessions.

The ups and downs of domestic violence are what make it so difficult for law enforcement personnel to get involved. They are not sure what is going right or wrong between couples until unfortunately, most times, it is too late. Our up-and-down, in-and-out relationship was also difficult for family, friends, and outsiders to understand. Vigorous corrective counseling needs to be directed so as to reach both partners.

I fasted and prayed for months that things would change and that the marriage would work. Finally, when I was asked to leave the last time, I resolved to get off the back-and-forth merry-go-round. Many more unpleasant things happened, but space does not permit their inclusion.

Abuse is being addressed here because it is so prevalent, misunderstood, and accepted. I could not believe that such a thing could happen in a marriage, especially to me. Studying about it and actually experiencing are like comparing night and day. Book knowledge does not begin to tell the story of abuse.

Abusers are unfortunately very hypocritical. They maintain a Dr. Jekyll-Mr. Hyde personality. They are very charming to people who don't know them, and they are very mean to their victims. Many of them unfortunately are also churchgoers and leaders. Perpetrators can easily influence the court system because they are so convincing. Few people believe the abused person. Abuse is tolerated in the church and society because few people really know what it is.

Personally I have friends who continue to endure abuse with ministers or church leaders. They are taught to endure suffering as bold soldiers. I have seen many of them constantly go up to the altar for prayer. They stand on the scripture, "Wives submit yourselves unto your own husbands, as it is fit in the Lord" Colossians 3:18. To them, leaving is never an option.

The couples either ignore or they do not read the very next verse: "Husbands, love your wives, and be not bitter against them" Colossians 3:19. "Husbands, love your wives, even as Christ also loved the church, and gave himself for it" Ephesians 5:25.

A good counselor is indispensable when couples are contemplating marriage. Counseling can expose abuse issues before lives are ruined. A close friend related her story to me. She was about to marry a man whose abuse was exposed. She called off the entire marriage, and he went his way.

Abusers rarely feel the need for counseling. I have heard of a few who obtained counseling, and their marriages were spared. One lady told her husband, "I simply cannot go on like this." He relented and went with her for the sessions.

Their marriage survived. Marriage should be an atmosphere where each person can grow as a nurtured flower in a fertile garden. The home should be a place where one can find peace and tranquility at any time, especially after a hard day's work. The apparent outside peace should exist inside.

While enduring a verbally abusive relationship, it was difficult to come home after an especially hard day at work. There was no one with which to communicate feelings and emotions. Having to attend weekly and Sunday night services were especially hard, being married to an abuser.

As we listen to the increased incidents of deaths of wives, children, and spouses, neighbors and others who knew them usually say, "They were nice people who kept to themselves." "We did see the cops over there a few times." In these times, sadly, few people know their neighbors anymore.

This information was never meant to be a clergy-bashing venture. Instead, the message here is that we need to pray for our leaders, the clergy, and their families. They are under tremendous pressures from many sources. Personal, family, and congregational issues place much responsibility on the ministers. Not all ministers and leaders are abusers. Many are very Godly and kind.

The plight of having to deal with these problems of self and others all the time places much stress on the ministers. Some were never called to the ministry by God. Some are not filled with the Holy Spirit, and as a result, they have no inner light and strength from which to draw to enable them help others.

Leaving the abuse arena was my decision after enduring certain repetitive behaviors for so long. I had endured verbal and physical abuse as a child, and the incidents of verbal battering had become all too frequent. While I cannot advise another woman to leave her marriage, I knew I had to get away from this abusive life, which to me was a second chapter of punishment.

With abuse, there are days when things seem as though they are going to be okay. This is why abuse is called cyclic. You find pleasant things to do and times to laugh. These are interspersed with intermittent times of battering. In my particular case, verbal battering persisted on a cyclic basis.

The old kiss-and-make up thing was a circus as far as I was concerned. A lot of couples thrive on abusing, being abused, and then enjoying the makeup times. Abuse has a way of destroying intimacy. If there is no love, everything is out of focus.

That morning before leaving the abuse, I lay in bed thinking about having to face another day with a congregation who thought our marriage was heavenly. I reflected on all the stormy Sunday mornings I had gone to church all dressed up and feeling terrible inside.

I had faithfully gone to church every service and even served as transportation on occasion for some of the members. I decided not to go that day, and I started a new chapter in my life. I could no longer be a hypocrite myself while I was pretending that all was well.

We had a local telecast that aired every Sunday morning and some Sunday nights during the abuse. Being raked over the coals before the telecasts was not an uncommon occurrence for me. I sang on the programs. Some people were critical of me without knowing what I was enduring.

The soundtracks were often delayed as I stood smiling at the camera while trying to look happy. Often people in the television audience can sense that something is wrong. When I see a telecast now, I can pick out women who are enduring abuse or some other negative things in other people's lives.

The perpetrator had left alone earlier to go to the church. While he was at church being his usual hypocritical self, I called a friend who suspected the abuse. Since he had recently told me to leave his house, I decided this would be the day and time I needed to leave the abuse forever.

Although I had never discussed the abuse with a coworker, she frequently voiced her knowledge of what I was going through. This friend and her family helped me to move to my own place about ten miles away. The perpetrator tried several times to lure me back, but enough was enough!

My prayer life had suffered due to the abuse. Now I could resume my life of prayer, fasting, and studying the Word. The constant ups and downs of abuse take their toll on one's personal as well as spiritual life and growth. Another bitter chapter of my life had closed. Later, we apologized for our parts in the breakup.

Domestic violence is a malady that is going nowhere anytime soon. It is a spiritual and unnatural stronghold ingrained in the fabric of life. It has been taught and shown by example for years. Vigorous early domestic violence education of youths needs to be somehow woven into the fabric of our society.

Just as with any other stronghold; the practice of domestic violence is a comfortable practice to those affected. It is learned behavior, just as eating sweets. We love to eat sweets although we know too many of them are bad for us. The merchants make lots of money, so sales will not stop.

Tolerance has been granted too long by partners and society. During my public health home visitation years, a lot of moms said that they discovered the father of their children was going to be an abuser. They forcefully (verbally and/or otherwise) got themselves out of the situation.

Some of the women were not aware of anything called abuse. They just determined that they would not be yelled at, talked down to, nor physically hurt in any way. Other women were so excited about having a man in their lives until they were willing to take anything any man dished out to them.

This brings up another issue regarding partner selection. I have met many Christian women who are praying for a man or a husband. They are practically willing to settle for any man just to have some companionship. Some are totally clueless to what is out there.

God has some very good men out there, but there are also some terrible prospects out there waiting for their chance to slither into the life of some sweet, naïve, unsuspecting, innocent partner. Again, I reiterate good counseling prior to marriage is indispensable.

Our present economy lends itself greatly to the practice of domestic violence. Abusers have low stress-tolerance levels. The slightest provocation sets them off. Loss of jobs, mortgage foreclosures, loss of possessions, and general disruption of the flow of life is very difficult for anyone.

Much has been written about abuse and violence. Many resources are available in your local community library. Safe shelters can be accessed by calling 1-800-ABUSE. We merely see the tip of the domestic abuse iceberg. Victims can be directed to the shelter nearest them.

The unfortunate thing about abuse is that children have to suffer needlessly, especially when they are not reached by a child protection agency. Children have uncanny ability to love their abusing parents, and a lot of the time they want to remain with them. Children will believe the abuser's lies.

Consider all of the red flags in a relationship before embarking on a lifetime venture with the person. Often what is wrong will not be corrected; it usually will get worse. As a rule, one adult cannot change the other to conform to your desire. What you see is not always what you get.

For ten years, I made excuses for the abuse. I had been warned early in marriage that the abuse would not stop without help. One evening, I received a call from someone in Orlando, Florida, who said she was a prophetess. She said I was being abused and should not remain in the situation.

I had no idea who she was and wondered how she got my number to call me. I remained in the abuse. I never found out who she was or if someone told her about my plight. I had to be convinced that leaving was the right thing to do. I thought about my oath at the altar and desired to honor it.

Being in an abusive situation was very confusing. The one who stood at the altar and vowed to protect me was abusing me. I never knew when an event was going to occur. Our home was supposed to be an example for the parishioners; instead, it was a hellacious house of unpredictable horrors.

Abused women are sometimes caught up in the "don't rock the boat" mentality. Abuse happens as long as you endure and allow it. It is somewhat like encountering a Dr. Jekyll and a Mr. Hyde all in the same day. You never know which personality you'll face, so you prepare for both.

One particular Sunday morning, we arrived at the abuser's pastorate. I had been raked over the coals all morning about some trivial matter. As we arrived at the church, the verbal abuse continued. Suddenly another sister arrived.

The abuser's personality and behavior did a complete about-face. He became very charming to the point that I wondered how such a behavior change could occur so quickly. Abusers are usually convincingly charming to those who don't know them.

Status is another reason the abused feel compelled to stay. We looked like the proverbial happy, successful couple. After all, he was a popular, successful pastor, and I was a nurse. We both had successful careers, made lots of money, had a nice big brick-front house, three automobiles, and a large camper. We both owned other properties.

People often say of the victim, "Why doesn't he or she get out of it?" Leaving is often danger filled because it threatens the perpetrator's well-being. Depending on his/her degree of violence, the victim may always be in danger. Some victims remain armed in case the perpetrator shows up.

The relationship is about power and control, and no abuser willingly relinquishes it. Restraining orders from the courts are only mild and often temporary deterrents to determined abusers. Restraining orders mainly serve as evidence that may be useful in court at a later date.

Many victims are constrained by economics. Abusers try to keep their victims either in debt or totally without financial resources so they cannot leave. She may wonder how she will be able to take care of herself and the kids if she leaves. Many women said they stayed because of the children.

Bible College had been placed on hold for a while during the abuse. My spouse brought various used and broken-down printers home for me to complete my homework. After a few times of having my homework either ink smeared or torn up by the printers, out of frustration, I stopped school for a while.

A former cherished classmate had completed Bible College and was enjoying a successful counseling practice. She found out why I had delayed my education and called me. She informed me that she had a word processor to give me. I went and picked up the processor. It had its own printer.

She told me to take the word processor and complete my Bible studies. She told me to keep the equipment as long as I needed it. I was able to complete the large volume of papers required by the College. Word processors were popular before computers were in wide use.

Graduation time came, and I was able to complete my specialist's degree in Christian counseling. I decided to delay my doctoral studies because of the abuse. Working and attending school was a bit much with the abuse. I did continue to play for Bible College functions and speak from time to time.

When the union was over, I entered graduate school for the doctoral degree. I changed to another College in the city and completed the course of study. The program was pretty intense and comprehensive. Graduation was completed, and I received my doctoral degree.

The loss of another union was both bitter and sweet, but I was comforted by the completion of my Bible studies. As I sat through the ceremony, I thought about the faithfulness of God and his love that allowed me to escape the abuse and to finally graduate from Bible College.

The Domestic Violence Section of the College has been strategically placed by God. He placed it in the heart of a registered nurse and professor to organize the institute. Domestic violence is a subject avoided by many leaders. It needs to be dealt with by all who are in training positions, leadership, and the clergy.

The school of DV could not have come at a more opportune time than when I was experiencing this dilemma. As stated earlier, my footsteps have indeed been ordered throughout my life. As you will see as you read, it appeared as if certain things just happened.

Nothing ever just happens, especially when you belong to the Lord. When you invite him as Lord over your life and affairs, he orchestrates events in your life. The perpetrators need much prayer. They need much counseling, but unless court ordered, many of them will never seek help.

Couples who are experiencing domestic violence need to reassess their relationships with God. With all of the hurt, rejection, and confusion, God is being left out. Abuse is a good position to be in to carelessly and accidentally lose one's soul.

Nurses are required to maintain credit education units in domestic violence to renew licenses biennially. Before seeing abuse up close, I had no idea of the magnitude of the problem despite the yearly trainings. When I saw an abused person at work, it was easy to go home and forget it. None of my training prepared me for an abusive lifestyle.

After seeing firsthand what abused people go through, I could empathize with them and work harder to get help for them. I became a better listener and advocate, whereas before, abuse was just some faraway topic. I have started keeping booklets and information for any abused person I happened to meet.

Abusers are very charming, as stated in another portion of this work. People usually don't believe the abused person is telling the truth. They only believe if they are in close contact with the couple or they actually witness the abuse. Abusers can convince people that they are very upstanding and harmless.

Going through abuse was not a pleasant experience, yet it endowed me with valuable knowledge and information to help other sufferers. The work supervisor who had been through abuse herself knew my situation immediately. As soon as the abuse started, she recognized what was happening.

She pointed it out to me and insisted that I get help. She allowed me to use accrued time and administrative leave to receive the help I needed. I could not believe I, of all people, had fallen into the trap of abuse. I tried to make the union work. I wanted to bond and have a perfect union.

When nurses and medical personnel see unexplained black eyes, broken limbs, and bruises in patients, abuse needs to be investigated. I have seen clients try to hide bruises under long sleeves and high collars. It is amazing the lengths victims will go to in order to protect their abusers.

People who abuse children and leave marks on them try to hide or cover up the evidence. Workers need to be vigilant at all times and report when injuries of either children or adults do not match their stories. Institutionalized clients also need to be monitored for abuse from some workers.

One respectable family in our church had a daughter who went to College. She became involved with an abuser, married him, and never completed her education. They got in a fight one Christmas morning, and she ended up in jail with him. She was very physically beautiful and talented and had great potential.

While in Bible College, we had a traveling professor who worked as a chaplain in the prison system. He said many women went to prison while trying to fight off or had killed an abusive mate. This professor also said a number of males were in prison for trying to protect their moms from abusive dads.

Some abusers are substance users which compounds the effects of the abuse. Sometimes partners are intimidated to the point of abetting or helping their mate commit crimes. They fear the abuser more than the consequences of the crime. I serviced two such clients during my career. Both went to jail.

MEDICAL NURSING

By the time I turned eighteen, I thought by now the statute of limitations on beatings for my latest offense had expired. Mother dear had mellowed, and I felt less threatened by her. My foster parents and I forgave each other for what happened, and we genuinely laughed together.

By now MD's health had started deteriorating. I hadn't started nurses' training yet, but I was still able to take her to the doctor and help her with her medications. I soon started nurses' training and was able to help her to understand a lot of what was wrong with her.

Medical nursing was the one area that first caught my attention. MD suffered with chronic high blood pressure. She also had diabetes with stasis ulcers, (rarely seen now) and later, congestive heart failure. The three hundred plus pounds she weighed for years were now taking their toll.

Blood pressure is the measure of the unit of force exerted against the wall of a blood vessel. It is the reading of what the heart is doing during its contracted, or active, phase and during its relaxed phase. Imagine water traveling through a hose.

The smaller the diameter of the inside of the hose, whether it is from blockage or any other reason, liquid cannot flow freely. Blood has difficulty flowing through narrowed blood vessels just as the water has problems flowing in the hose. Such pressure reads as high on a measuring device.

High blood pressure is known as the silent killer because it is often without symptoms. If there is a family history of high blood pressure, one needs to keep an eye on the pressure, watch salt intake, and get under the care of a good physician. Do not neglect prayer by all means.

Many people walk around with high blood pressure never feeling a thing, until one day a stroke occurs. If you are taking medication, do so until your healing is confirmed by your doctor. Continue to eat sensibly and avoid stressors as much as possible. Know your cholesterol and other lab numbers.

Cholesterol is a fatty substance that causes plaque to build up in one's arteries. The cholesterol needs to be controlled with prayer, medications, low-fat diet, exercise, and again avoidance of stress. Plaque can block blood vessels in the brain and heart, causing irreversible damage.

God's overshadowing presence as well as one's faith plays a significant role in healing. Healing is a miraculous supernatural experience that happens, which medical science cannot explain. My first book *Natural Bread Is Not Enough* addresses some of my own personal healings.

Obesity is very prevalent and often accepted in our society today. Obese people were used in the movie industry in the past as the subjects of humor. Beauty pageants for obese women are not uncommon today. Attractive clothing now comes in extra-large sizes to accommodate obese people.

Obesity leads to many of the chronic illnesses such as high blood pressure, heart trouble, high cholesterol, diabetes, and a myriad of ailments that can lead to an early death. When physical education was taken from the school curriculum, pretty soon, an epidemic of obesity followed.

Thanks to the first lady of America's focus on prevention, obesity is being sensibly addressed. Actions are being taken among our youths to stem the tide of another generation of overweight people. Camps designed specifically for addressing the problems of childhood obesity now exist.

Diabetes is a condition in which a cluster of cells, known as the islets of Langerhans, in the pancreas is not working properly. Starches cannot be properly broken down, and they become sugars in the body. With my new knowledge, I was able to help MD plan her diet. MD's husband, Daddy B. was mainly healthy until he developed gout, a form of arthritis. MD loved all of the soul foods, and she could lay out a feast that would please any king. She fed Daddy B. and me very well. Although Mother dear was obese, obesity was rare at that time.

Coming back to see my foster parents was therapeutic for all of us. We became the best of friends. Precious time and years were lost during those years I was gone. As a child, I did not know how to communicate my feelings about the perceived wrongful beatings.

I later learned that my leaving had left a gaping hole in Daddy B.'s heart. He had big dreams for his little girl, and I aborted them by running away. Running away may solve the immediate dilemma, but it creates future problems. It gets us out of the fiery arena, but the consequences await us later.

I, along with MD, Daddy B., and my own aunt, were able to coexist peacefully the rest of their lives. We were able to forgive and forget. As I completed high school, married, and later entered College, these parents continued to support me emotionally.

Despite all of the hard feelings, misunderstandings, and brokenness, we were able to salvage our lives and move on. My foster mom gave me a lovely yard wedding when I got married. Daddy B. stood tall with pride as he gave me away. They both showed how proud of me they were with every accomplishment I made.

For several years during my marriage, my foster parents were there for me. When we celebrated Mother's Day and Father's Day at our church, they came and stood proudly as my parents. We bought each other greeting cards and gifts for holidays. Life was good.

When we do not forgive and clear the air, it is sort of like packing garbage into our bodies and minds and holding on to it. Eventually we are so full of garbage until we cannot think objectively or live our lives peacefully and to the fullest. For Bible believers, those who believe in heaven, just forget about going there.

During my childhood years, there was always someone near or around us who had some chronic illness. Watching the sick person always caused me to want to do something for them. When other kids at school developed a nose bleed or other problems, it concerned me.

Older people always knew how to pull out home remedies to solve a lot of illnesses. Home remedies were relied upon more than doctor visits. My own MD kept her own arsenal of remedies. Castor oil and/or chicken soup were the biggest weapons in the arsenal.

Castor oil was given for the common cold, tummy aches, and just about everything else. Various teas were given for some ailments. If the illness was not cured with remedies, then people were taken to the doctor. Some illnesses were self-limiting. Aspirin was another big panacea.

When I developed rubeola, or red measles, my foster mom recognized it immediately and took me to the doctor. Her aunt made some sort of tea, which she said caused the rash to complete its cycle.

Having been taken to the doctor when MD first got me, I received all of the immunizations available at that time. A nurse came to our school and gave every one of us our smallpox shot. Somehow I escaped getting the chicken pox and mumps.

Control of Communicable Diseases in Man by Abram S. Benenson is highly recommended reading for a comprehensive review of all communicable diseases. It is updated periodically and may be purchased where medical books are purchased, such as a College bookstore.

Prior to the development of the immunizations, loss of life to communicable diseases was rampant. Some parents will not allow their children to be immunized because they cannot stand to subject their child to the pain of the shots. These communicable diseases can lead to death.

As an industrialized country, we are not as up to par with immunizations as we should be. As a result, some of the old diseases are still around. Smallpox killed many people, but with the advent of the vaccine, it was basically eradicated. Parents are encouraged to immunize their children.

As I watched various illnesses and experienced them myself, I resolved that one day I would be able to do something about all of the sickness and suffering. In some cases, just being with the patient and emotionally supporting them was a valuable tool. Listening to them vent their feelings also helped.

When my mother-in-law was dying of a brain tumor, I stayed with her while she was waiting for the surgeon. Just carrying her belongings and talking and listening to her meant a lot, which she later verbalized to me. She eventually succumbed.

People who travel internationally need to be aware of their potential exposure to and possible transmission of communicable diseases. Check with your local public health department regarding necessary immunizations prior to traveling. Clinics known as Fast Track are now a part of most health departments.

Waiting times for immunizations at Fast Track clinics are fairly short, and moms can be on their way. The child should have a primary care or regular physician for physicals. At the Fast Track clinic, children will be immunized if they are not ill or running any temperature.

Adults need to keep up to date on their tetanus shots also. When cuts and bruises occur, such as in an auto accident, if tetanus has not been received within five to ten years, you may receive one at this time. Tetanus is known familiarly as lock jaw.

When natural disasters occur, people are often at risk for tetanus due to cuts and bruises caused by debris. You may also receive a tetanus shot prior to surgical intervention. Stab or puncture wounds contaminated with soil or infectious material can introduce the tetanus spores into the body.

After a few years of fellowship with my foster parents, illnesses began to take their toll on them. Daddy B. developed painful gout in his joints, which quickly plunged him into a wheelchair. He could not endure the pain or the loss of independence. He never ceased being a macho man.

Gout is an inherited metabolic disturbance that has to do with the body's ability to excrete uric acid. The disorder resembles arthritis in that it produces joint pain with redness and swelling. The pain is usually felt in the first joint of the great toe, then later in other joints of the foot and/or body.

Little was known about gout, and therefore Daddy B. suffered great pain. Although he was gentle and often perceived as henpecked, he was very strong and masculine. Gout proved to be too much for him, and he quickly gave up the will to live. He passed away within six months of the diagnosis.

After Daddy B. passed away, MD began to grieve and was also gone within less than two years of his death. The night she passed away had been preceded by a day of preparation for her relatives to visit. Several out-of-town cousins had called and told her they were coming to see her for her birthday.

MD spent all day Saturday cooking her favorite soul food dishes for her family. These foods were the worst she could have prepared for herself, and they included: fried chicken, collard greens cooked in ham hocks, seasoned rice, macaroni and cheese, fresh green beans, cake, and pie.

The relatives telephoned near dark and disappointed MD by saying they couldn't make the trip. MD helped herself to the soul food. She became very ill and was rushed to the hospital, where she passed away. I traveled the thirty miles, but she had passed before I arrived.

Now that my foster parents were gone, I began to reflect on my years with them. I felt some guilt because of my running away years ago. Then I thought of the times we spent together after the reunion. Those good years gave me consolation and made me feel happy that we had reunited.

A person's death is difficult to accept if you did not do all you could for them. MD had left detailed instructions with her lawyer and the executrix regarding her will and funeral plans. She had left the planning of her funeral to me because she felt I would carry out her wishes.

Her aunt wasn't too pleased, but we managed to get through everything with little friction. MD had meted out her belongings fairly, which caused everyone to be pleased that they at least got something they didn't already have. We all parted in peace.

This would have been my last year of nurses' training from the associate's degree program. I had looked forward to the day when both parents would see me march down those aisles and receive my diploma. I felt sad that death took them before I graduated.

Somehow I planned the services, took care of MD's necessary business, and got through the time of grief. I returned to College and quickly became reabsorbed into my studies. The chapter of my foster parents was closed in my life.

We need to treat people as if every day is our last with them. It is not always easy, but we should try. Time lost in bad vibes and bad actions toward others can never be regained. If you have trouble forgiving someone, ask God to help you.

Learning the various illnesses and their treatments during medical-surgical nursing gave me the information I needed to help people in my community as well as in the hospital. The information came a little late to help my parents. Preventive information would have helped, had I known it.

Elderly people had a saying that makes sense now. They would say, "An ounce of prevention is worth a pound of cure." They meant it was easier to prevent some disease, disorder, or any problem than it was to cure it. Try getting rid of belly fat or obesity overnight without liposuction.

I could have explained to MD that her heart was a muscular organ. Those heart muscles were like rubber bands that could be stretched by her heart having to pump so hard over the years. The high pressures and the weight caused the heart muscles to lose their elasticity and fail as a pump.

Over a period of time, the heart muscles were stretching until they could stretch no more. Congestive heart failure was MD's final diagnosis. When the heart fails to be able to pump blood through the vessels to other organs and systems, life ceases.

When nurses graduated in the past, we were required to take the Nightingale pledge as written below. It was composed by an instructor at Harper Hospital in Detroit, Michigan, in the 1800s. It somewhat follows the pattern of the oath which physicians were required to take, known as the Hippocratic Oath.

The Nightingale Pledge

I solemnly pledge myself, before God and in the presence of this assembly, to pass my life in purity and to practice my profession faithfully.
I will abstain from whatever is deleterious and mischievous and will not take or knowingly administer any harmful drug. I will do all in my power to maintain and elevate the standard of my profession and will hold in confidence all personal matters committed to my keeping and all family affairs coming to my knowledge in the practice of my calling.
With loyalty, I will endeavor to aid the physician in his work and devote myself to the welfare of those committed to my care.

Nurses were expected to be women of good character and impeccable standards. This should be the hallmark of every profession. There is something called bedside manner. It is the method by which we deliver services to our bed-bound clients. In recent years, bedside manner has been less than desirable by some in the profession.

As professionals, we must deliver what we would like to have delivered to us. There are times when we may find ourselves on the receiving end of the care system. Make it a point to deliver the kind of care you would desire to receive. Good manners should prevail in every care situation.

There is nothing more frightening and disconcerting to clients than to have staff standing around discussing them as if they were objects. Whispered comments should never be made about clients. Include them in what is being discussed about them.

Bedside walking rounds were once popular at the beginning and end of working shifts in the hospital. The purpose of the rounds was to brief the oncoming staff about the clients and their orders, medications, and care regime.

Include clients as much as possible in their own care. Inform them what you plan to do before doing it. Help them become familiar with what medications they are getting. Be kind to family and visitors. Include family when possible.

SURGICAL NURSING

When medical procedures cannot reach a problem, surgical intervention may be necessary to correct the problem. My first surgical experience occurred in the surgeon's office where I worked as a young adult. I was encouraged to pursue a nursing career.

The surgeon gave me permission to watch surgical procedures in his office. Minor surgical procedures where general anesthesia was not required were performed by this doctor several times a week in his office. I was taught a lot about preoperative and postoperative care.

The surgeon operated at the local hospital in the mornings and saw his postoperative clients in the afternoons in his office. I was given the opportunity to cleanse and dress wounds, remove surgical drains, and remove surgical sutures.

Application of plaster casts for fractures was a frequent procedure in the doctor's office. I was taught and allowed to assist in applying them to broken limbs. Learning how to spot a circulation problem was part of the training.

The time came when I had to have surgery. As all women should be doing monthly, I had been carefully examining my breasts for abnormalities and lumps. One day, while I was palpating for lumps, I discovered something deeply embedded beneath the skin.

The fear of possible breast cancer gripped me. This growth was about the size of a thick dime. At first I was afraid to tell anyone, especially the surgeon. The thought of having a flat chest at my age was unthinkable. The surgeon said he would check the lump when all of the clients were finished.

In fear, I left before the doctor could get to me. The nurse called me at home to inquire as to why I had left. I tearfully told her my fears. She encouraged me to come back the next day. I was consumed with the thought of having to have surgery and possible mastectomy.

I had seen clients in the office who had the surgery, and it scared me. The next afternoon the surgeon asked if I were willing to allow two flabs of fat to take seventy-five years off my life. He examined me and informed me that I needed to check into the hospital for a biopsy and possible mastectomy.

I felt like everything was spiraling out of control and it was curtains for me. Before I was fully awake from the anesthesia, I kept trying to feel the bandages to see if my chest was flat. The thick bandages kept me in suspense.

Finally the surgeon came around. He assured me that everything was fine. The biopsy had proved to be negative, and I only had a lumpectomy. Mammography was not a routine test then. Ladies, take advantage of this diagnostic tool along with your own personal self-breast monthly examination.

A negative biopsy gave me a feeling of relief. I began to appreciate the fear women feel when told they have a breast lump. This is one of those instances where an ounce of prevention is worth a pound of cure. Ladies, make sure you are diligent about the (SBE) self-breast examination.

After years of the seemingly rough manhandling during mammography exams, I skipped it a few times. I declined all the mashing, squeezing, and pinching of the test. My excuse and attitude was that if there is nothing wrong with this part of my anatomy, it surely will be with years of this type of handling.

Finally my allergy physician's nurse backed me in a corner about missing the exams. I told her why I had missed the exams. The nurse put me in touch with a precision-imaging mammography center. The exam was quick, painless, and my results came back in a very timely manner.

The centers cater to the needs of women. After being tested at this center, my fears and dread of the examination ceased. It was called a digital imaging center. The cost was no more than any other mammography center. My insurance paid everything.

The obituary section of the newspapers still unfortunately reports too many young women dying of breast cancer. Our local city has very strong breast cancer advocacy programs. There is also a very strong support system for the survivors where I currently reside.

Men have breast cancer, but not nearly as frequently as women. Education, surveillance, early detection, and early intervention are still our best tools for eradicating this dreaded entity from the earth. All women should learn how to do self-breast exams and be diligent about doing them.

Locally, the breast awareness center also encourages a buddy system, which is helpful. When we feel we are not alone in something, the whole process is bearable. The nursing staff of your doctor's office can teach you how to do self-breast exams. Always report any abnormalities to your doctor.

After training, I spent time working on a surgical floor and in the surgical intensive care unit. When I had surgery, it gave me a chance to see and understand what surgery is like for other people. Spirometry and repositioning are done postoperatively to prevent pneumonia.

A plastic device called a spirometer is used in the spirometry breathing treatments. Clients are encouraged to become mobile as quickly as possible to prevent the long-term complications of bed rest (i.e., pneumonia, blood clots, constipation, decubitus ulcers).

The surgical area of nursing brought back memories of the instructions I had received while working for the surgeon. Instead of remaining in surgical nursing, I chose to explore all of the other areas of nursing. Most of my career was spent in the area of public health and pediatrics.

As a nursing student in the baccalaureate program, we were all required to rotate through each area of nursing. While going through the surgical rotation, we had to choose a preoperative family. We were required to interview and follow the client preoperatively, interoperatively, and postoperatively.

My case consisted of two brothers who were going to have surgery simultaneously. One brother had kidney failure. His brother was donating one of his kidneys to him. This happened during the years when kidney transplantation and dialysis were new procedures.

One doctor who was connected with our College had just invented a sports drink. Since my clients were renal patients, I had to become familiar with the anatomy and physiology of the kidney and dialysis. At the time, there were two types of dialysis: peritoneal and renal. My surgical client would have had to have renal dialysis.

Dialysis is a process by which the blood is cleansed of impurities because the person's kidneys cannot do it. We can live with one operating kidney; however, when both of the kidneys are absent, poisons build up in the body, and life soon ceases.

Uncontrolled high blood pressure and diabetes are two examples of diseases that can eventually lead to renal or kidney failure. Dialysis centers are located in cities throughout the USA where clients go approximately two to three times a week to have the waste removed from their bloodstream.

One brother's kidneys had failed. Without a transplant or lifelong dialysis, he faced death. The brothers made the decision to have the surgery. On the day of surgery, I, along with the surgical team, scrubbed up and prepped for the surgery. Each brother was prepped in a separate operating room.

One surgical team removed the kidney for the donor while the other surgical team removed the brother's diseased kidneys. Once the healthy kidney was removed from the donor, it was placed in a normal saline solution and carried in to the recipient's surgical room.

I was expecting the kidney to be placed into the back of the client where normal kidneys lie. Instead, transplanted kidneys are placed into an area of rich blood supply in the abdominal area. The kidney was a perfect match. Both brothers resumed their normal lives afterward.

I offer a final note on staff decorum: Conversation over anesthetized and/or comatose clients needs to be spoken with care. It did not occur with this client, but I have been told by clients that they heard everything said about them while they were supposedly "out of it."

Before "out of body" experiences were widely known, televised, and discussed, several clients told me things they saw and heard while they were supposedly "out of it," or they were going through some procedure to revive them. The information was later confirmed.

Psychiatric Nursing

There will be no attempts to address the history of psychiatry or to write about all of the various psychiatric disorders. This writing will limit itself mainly to the experiences and encounters of one psychiatric nurse. Only the disorders encountered will be addressed.

We live in a computer age, where anyone has access to the Internet. Psychiatric information is readily available at one's fingertips. Medical and other libraries also provide more current information. Treatment modalities are also ever changing.

Psychiatric nursing is indeed an area where dedicated workers are much in demand. With our open society, people can walk around appearing to lead normal lives. These same people may be on the brink of a breakdown. In today's economy, many are living on the edge.

How many times have we listened to the evening news reports of people seen as nice and normal by their neighbors? Yet those same nice people turn up in the news as committing some awful acts. Was this the act of a sane mind?

With the advent of new living standards and drugs and substance misuse, "normal" behavior is difficult to define anymore. Identifiable psychiatric illnesses do exist. Medication and treatment have caused those needing help to blend very easily into society.

As will be discussed later in this writing, people could easily be committed to mental health facilities on unfounded information in the past. In today's society, one has to have proof of the person's insanity. Law officials and medical health professionals must now be consulted in order for a person to be institutionalized.

According to legal history, a lady by the name of Maxine Baker was responsible for initiating the Baker Act of 1971 in Florida. This act allows for involuntary and temporary commitment of a person to a mental facility.

There must be proof that the person has a mental illness, is self-neglectful, or is capable of harming himself or others.

The psychiatric nurse must possess good observation and reporting skills. In our psychiatric rotation, we were taught to do what was known as process recordings. We were required to record all of our verbal and physical interactions over a given period of time.

Behavior patterns whether normal or aberrant could be determined after studying the recordings over a period of time. These were helpful in guiding the psychiatrist in his treatment of the client.

Clients' families should always be considered in the care of psychiatric illnesses. Psychiatric illnesses seem to affect the cohesiveness of the family. There is blame and finger-pointing as to whose side of the family the problem originated. The families also struggle with feelings of guilt.

Psychiatric nursing deals with the treatment and care of the mentally challenged population. Before the Baker Act was instituted, people could be committed to a mental institution without being formerly diagnosed as mentally ill.

If a family member had some strange behavior or they acted a bit eccentric, they were deemed as one who needed to be committed to an institution away from the rest of the family. Normal, nonassertive people ended up being placed against their will.

Mental illness was also thought to be caused by a person being possessed of the devil. The mentally ill or those thought to be off-balance were locked away as animals and treated with cruelty. They had no rights. Families hid their mentally ill relatives away from public scrutiny.

One popular question that once appeared on important papers such as job applications, medical histories, etc. was "Is there a history of insanity in your family?" There was once a general aura of humor regarding the mentally ill person. Mental illness is no laughing matter. It wreaks untold havoc on those afflicted.

Much has been done to recognize mental illness as a disease just as any other illness. It is treatable to the point that people can function normally in society. Much still needs to be done in improving the way we treat this population.

My nursing interests never led me into the psychiatric arena. In the days when nurses were floated to hospital areas to balance staffing, I worked on some psychiatric units. During those days, clients were sedated with drugs such as Haldol, lithium, Thorazine, Mellaril, or some other strong medications.

These strong medications rendered the clients almost helpless. Clients walked around with a zombie-like appearance due to the medications. Other clients were tied in bed with jacket or body restraints. I have seen clients pick the restraints totally loose very quickly while in a manic state.

Medication strengths are now adjusted to the clients' needs. Other medications that eliminate the extrapyramidal symptoms are now being used. Many people now function quite well in society with their medications. Even some movie stars have written of their illnesses being controlled by medications.

Clients suffering from delirium tremors or drug withdrawal were sent to the psychiatric ward before drug rehabilitation centers were popular. Any entity that did not fit into the ordinary medical picture seems to have been sent to the psychiatric ward.

The elderly clients who manifested any symptoms of dementia were sent to the psychiatric ward. Sometimes kids who ran away from home ended up in the psychiatric ward. It seemed few regular hospitals knew exactly who to classify as mentally ill or where to put them.

A close encounter with a psychiatric client occurred some years ago in my own home. A household member at that time had begun to talk about seeing Martin Luther King, John F. Kennedy, and Robert Kennedy. All of these men were dead at the time. The man was convinced he saw these three men.

I had already graduated from College and was working a night shift at the local hospital. My psychiatric training was behind me, and I did not connect the experience I was about to encounter as a psychiatric one. This sighting of the dead men was indeed strange. I wondered if he were just having dreams.

A number of other strange behaviors occurred which puzzled me, but I still did not connect any of the behavior as being of a psychiatric nature. Then one day, I was doing something inside my home when I heard the noise of a crowd approaching. I ran to the front window and looked outside.

From my front window I saw a humongous crowd of people heading toward our home. A police officer in a squad car was riding alongside the crowd, and this person was leading the crowd. He was both preaching and uttering profanities at the same time.

He had just had a confrontation with some lady and knocked her flat on the streets. Since his behavior was so erratic, someone who knew him called an officer. As he started walking home, a crowd of people who knew him followed to see what would happen.

The officer pulled into our driveway as I met him. He said, "Ma'am, you need to get this man to a psychiatrist as soon as possible and get him medicated. The crowd listened intently to every word, and then they dispersed. The officer left, and I was left alone to deal with a bipolar case.

I was so in the middle of the forest until I could not see the trees, so to speak. I called a psychiatric doctor and explained what the officer had told me to do. The doctor was able to see the man immediately. He was started on medication, and his behavior eventually began to improve.

After a time on the medication, this man stopped taking it without my knowledge. He did not like the side effects of the medications. When he was off the medication, his behavior was maniacal. One night, he tried to drive his truck into a tent revival in progress. No one was hurt.

My life changed drastically. The man's family began to blame me. One of his older brothers verbally attacked me and said, "I hear you have let our brother just run the streets." "You need to control him." This was hard to deal with because the man was grown, and I was responsible for him.

We went through several months of stressful events because of the on-and-off medication routine. When a loved one is experiencing a horrific event, it is difficult to be objective about it. Only in retrospect can one realize what should have been done in the situation. Denial worked for a time.

There are times when we walk through unpleasant places alone. Prayer and the word are indispensable. "When thou passest through the waters, I will be with thee; and through the rivers, they shall not overflow thee: when thou walkest through the fire, thou shall not be burned" Isaiah 43:2.

Being a nurse was of little comfort to me. Had I been taking care of someone out of the home, coping would have been easier. The symptoms happened so insidiously until I totally missed them. The man was able to function like a normal person between episodes of mania.

Diagnosing was not my job, but I should have been able to recognize the symptoms. After all, I had been trained in psychiatric nursing. After all of that training, I did not expect my first psychiatric experience would be in my house. Being so close to the problem made it hard to intervene objectively.

One night, before going to a Western state, the man came home around midnight. He had been taking his medication, and I began to have a feeling that things would be okay after all. He wanted me to sit down and listen because he wanted to talk about what had happened to him earlier in the evening.

I sat down and listened intently. He talked calmly and rationally. He said that as he was driving along, a voice told him to go and park his car over a grave which he did. He said the voice gave him other instructions, which he followed.

I recognized the problem, and I knew I had to get consistent help for him. I convinced him to come to the psychiatrist's office the next day. Thankfully, he was exhausted, and we made it through the night. Surprisingly, he quietly went to the psychiatrist. Medications were restarted in the form of injections every three months.

The man was able to function at his printing shop job for a time. He was a favorite of his elderly female boss who owned and operated the shop. Up until now, he had been a good employee, so she tolerated his behavior. Between episodes of mania, the man was able to function normally and talk rationally.

By the end of the year, one of the man's brothers who lived in the West invited us to come out there. He thought his brother could get better medical care. We locked up the house and asked the neighbor's to keep an eye on things. We left some family members in charge of the other belongings.

We then flew out West. I felt greatly relieved with the change of environment. The West was so pleasant and sunny, and the people were so nice. We lived with this family while the man received treatment.

We immediately connected with a Baptist church, where I played for one of the choirs. The man received excellent care at the county charity hospital. They helped him to learn a new job skill which he was able to do five days a week. Pretty soon, he was stabilized on the medication.

Being out West was so different. Finally I had someone who could be objective to talk to about the problem. People were so supportive and understanding. God always knows what we need and when we need it. If we trust him, he places us in circumstances that are best for us.

The church and the community of these people's friends reached out to help in every way they could. I loved the Western weather, environment, and the people. I thought this would be a good place to settle down when the present problems were resolved.

It was easy for me to get a job at a government hospital. I did not have to meet the reciprocity requirements because this was a government institution. The salary was great. I went through the rigorous and intense twelve-week orientation. The orientation honed in on sharpening hands-on nursing skills.

While at the government hospital, I met nurses from all over the world as well as the United States. We worked well together and had a lot of fun. I had never seen such long hospital halls. I wore out a new pair of heavy-duty nurses; shoes in three months with the rigorous work schedule.

One night, the man's dad telephoned very late. He sounded inebriated, and he wanted to speak to his son. The son who was the patient acted as if the call really upset him. He requested to go back to the South immediately. He gave as an excuse that someone wanted him to preach.

Truth was, the man had left a girlfriend with their young child back home, and she wanted him to come back. I did not know about his connection with the lady nor their child.

We saw no rest until we made plans for him to go back to the South. I resigned from the government hospital, and we rode a Greyhound bus back to home.

After returning home, eventually the man was no longer in my home, nor was he my responsibility. I was able to go on with my career and business freely. After that psychiatric experience, I decided to leave the psychiatric arena forever. My real desire was to work with children.

For a time, I went back to the local community hospital. I worked on a general medical floor most of the time. There was very little demand for a pediatrics ward. The sicker kids got transferred thirty-plus miles away to the teaching hospital. The others spent time on the lesser-sick adult wards.

Since it was a small hospital, nurses had to float to various areas to satisfy staffing quotas. I was never sure where I would be working from day to day. I was floated through medical, surgical, labor and delivery, postpartum, nursery, ICU, and the medical floor, which also housed psychiatry.

Night shifts were generally readily available, which made it easy for me to get a job immediately. No one wanted to work night shifts. Night shifts paid a differential, which meant more income. This also allowed me to attend church freely on Sundays.

The medical floor usually housed patients with an assortment of illnesses. Among them were genuine medical patients, psychiatric clients, and the overflow from other units. The orientation at the Western government hospital had well prepared me for the challenges of caring for such a varied group.

There was another unit that housed an eighteen-bed open ward. Elderly men and women were placed on the ward mainly because many of them were not alert or aware of where they were. Only a curtain surrounding the beds separated each person.

My assignments ranged from working these two wards to labor and delivery or the newborn nursery. When premature deliveries occurred at night, the babies were quickly sent to the nearby teaching hospital. Such varied assignments required a high degree of flexibility and willingness to float.

In those days, I was just grateful to have a job, making more money than I had ever made. I was surrounded by former schoolmates, a neighbor who was an LPN, and other friendly staff. This made the job very pleasant and the nights pass quickly.

A lot of the clients slept through the night. Others usually required every-four-hour medications, dressing changes, gastric or nasogastric tube feedings, intravenous medications, or respiratory percussions. Respiratory therapists were available for other breathing treatments.

The psychiatric clients who were housed on the medical floor were pretty well sedated by the time I came on the eleven-to-seven night shift. Occasionally someone with delirium tremors stayed awake and acted out. Other clients with dementia became noisy or acted out in some way.

In those days, every client got a light sponge bath and back rub before being tucked in for the night. Just about everyone also got a sleeping pill. Every client also received a morning bed bath unless they could bathe themselves. Caseloads were not as heavy as today's assignments.

Nurses had time to attend to the clients' needs. Recently, I visited a hospitalized friend, and I was appalled at the heavy caseloads and staff responsibilities. It is a wonder anyone gets any quality care. It seems it took hours of ringing the call bell before my friend was able to get any help.

Taking care of mentally challenged citizens in a hospital setting was not as difficult and threatening as caring for them in one's home. This experience helped me to be able to empathize with families who have mentally challenged family members.

Some years ago, a biological family member of mine received a gunshot wound to the head. It left him mentally challenged. He functioned much like the patient I cared for up close. He lived with a strong positive family member who was able to deal with him. He has tried her patience and lost.

Having attended a two-year nursing associate's degree program and a four-year BS psychiatric nursing program allowed me the benefit of having two separate rotations of training. My first psychiatric rotation took place in a private mental facility. Only wealthy clients were treated there.

The facility was situated on several sprawling acres in the countryside. The lawn, shrubbery, and trees appeared to be manicured. This facility had been a country club at one time. There was a relaxed atmosphere, and there were fewer clients than a regular state hospital.

Clients had private sessions, group sessions, and family counseling sessions. Their identities and their personal information were carefully guarded, just as all clients' information should be held in confidentiality. Clients were always well dressed in fashionable casual attire.

We were taught how to identify the various types of mental illnesses and their therapeutic regimes. We were also taught healthy ways to conduct healthy interpersonal interactions with the clients. The facility had more of an air of sophistication than of a psychiatric hospital.

No one seemed to ever be in any lockup rooms. Had this been my only psychiatric experience, I would have had a skewed view of psychiatry. Clients seemed to rarely have outbursts or acting-out experiences. The physicians always appeared relaxed to me in comparison to the other facility.

My second psychiatric rotation took place at one of the state mental institutions. There were far more clients, and the place was noisier. Some clients required lockup. This time, the sprawling landscape looked like a large school campus. There was sparse lawn and shrubbery, and it was not as green as the private place.

The clients' attire ranged from looking like rag dolls to being neatly dressed. It was recreation time at the facility, and the grounds were practically crowded with people. There were therapists and other workers out with their clients. As students, we had each been assigned a new client each week.

Our function was to stay with the client and observe the behavior. We had been given a certain case such as schizophrenia, which we had to identify and learn the symptoms. The interaction was written up and discussed in our group sessions.

We were taught which medications and therapies would likely be used in each disorder. There seemed to be more electroshock therapies than in the private hospital, perhaps because the population was larger. This treatment was popularly used at one time to break up severe depression.

In addition to their treatment regime, clients had daily routines of scheduled activities to allay apathy and lethargy. None of the psychiatric training prepared me for what I experienced in my own personal life. There was no ABC manual or set of instructions for use with in one's household.

Being intimately involved in a psychiatric case up close, allowed me to be able to empathize with other families. People with mental illnesses can lead normal lives when they follow their regime of treatment. Those who are kept bathed in prayer and in the word also get along better.

When a family has to deal with mental illness, it can be very frustrating and draining. Families who find that they are dealing with affected relatives need to avail themselves to as much family counseling as possible. Arm yourselves with as much information as possible. Seek respite to retain your own sanity.

Hours become days when dealing with mentally challenged loved ones. Things are very blurred until you step away from the problem and look at it from a distance. The relative mentioned previously, the one with the head wound, wanted to come and live with me. Past experience made me decline his offer.

He smoked marijuana, which complicated his condition. At times, he was a sweet loving, charming son, and other times he was out of control. Only one strong, assertive, positive relative was able to deal with him. He pulled capers on weaker family members. He was very manipulative.

Recently when his mom died, he was invited to live with another relative. For months, he took his medicine and did well. He decided to test the waters one day. Instead of paying his room and board with his income, he took all of his money and went on a trip.

He disregarded the relative and expected to get by with the same manipulative behavior that worked for him in the past. When he returned home, this relative had set all of his belongings outside and would not allow him access to her residence again.

Somehow he made peace with this relative, atoned for his mistake, and was taken back into the home. He has rigid limits set for him and rules he must follow if he is to remain in her household. This young fellow has done well with the tough love and consistent environment.

Psychiatric nursing has its work well mapped out in these times of a recession. People who would ordinarily get along well are being pressed to the brink due to multiple losses of jobs, homes, and possessions. The social service providers are running out of resources.

Natural disasters seem to have proliferated, which drive people to the brink. Sudden losses without resources to rebuild their lives leaves people devastated. Without an anchor such as the word and the Lord's help, people have no way of coping.

A televangelist once told of a woman who came to his tent crusade. She requested prayer for her sister who was in a psychiatric hospital. He blessed a handkerchief and sent it to the sister who got well.

Prayer is a powerful force that is most often overlooked in our efforts to succeed in life. It is usually our last resort. The lady who had the evangelist to pray for her sister through the prayer handkerchief took her leading from the book of Acts in the King James Version of the Bible.

"And God wrought special miracles by the hands of Paul: so that from his body were brought unto the sick handkerchiefs or aprons, and the diseases departed from them, and the evil spirits went out of them" Acts 19:11-12. Paul was doing the works Christ had said believers would do.

Paul the apostle was the man in scripture who arrested many of God's people and made havoc of their churches. One day, he was on his way to Damascus to persecute the church. He had first gone to the high priest to obtain letters to legally do the wrong that he was already doing.

On his way to Damascus, Paul, whose name was Saul at the time, had a supernatural experience with the Lord that changed him forever. After this experience, the Lord changed Saul's name to Paul. The book of Acts captures Paul's life and ministry.

This experience caused him to become convinced of the authenticity of Christ. Acts chapter 9 captures Paul's story about his conversion from a church persecutor to an advocate for the church and its people. Paul was credited with writing two-thirds of the New Testament.

The power of God from his body was transferred to the handkerchiefs and aprons. When they were placed on the bodies of people, they received healing. This belief is held in charismatic and Pentecostal circles even today. The lady at the crusade believed and received.

As students of psychiatric nursing, we were required to watch the movie *The Three Faces of Eve*. It seems that more than one personality was operating through the lady one at a time and causing her behavior to manifest whatever personality happened to be present at the time.

In psychiatry, a number of unusual phenomena do occur. In Pentecostal and charismatic circles unusual phenomena also sometimes occur. We live in a world where everything is not always what it appears. We need to be balanced where supernatural experiences are present.

As school kids, we found it easy to watch the magicians and be awed at their tricks. We always remembered the tricks, but we never questioned by what method the tricks truly came about. I often reflect back on the day the magician with the light bulb prophesied that I would never be a nurse.

It would have been comforting if someone had told me I would experience the things I went through—especially the psychiatric ones. "And we know all things work together for good to them that love God, to them who are called according to his purpose" Romans 8:28.

Maternal
and Child Health

When we think of maternal and child health, we formulate mental pictures of moms affectionately interacting with their babies. Mom has birthed her baby with no complications. There is a dad somewhere in the picture, and all is well in their world.

Somewhere in the other picture is another woman whose arms and womb long to hold a baby. A great majority of women marry or remain single, conceive and birth babies. They are totally oblivious to the fact that there are other women who just cannot produced a child from their bodies.

Some women spontaneously abort or they never conceive, and the sheer pleasure of cradling and caressing their own baby never happens. Still there are others who bring forth a special needs child, and the parents can never carry out the plans they might have had for their baby.

When the author had been diagnosed as a mother to be, there was much excitement in the air. I went to the campus infirmary, as I was still in College. They ran the test and called home to notify my husband of the test results. In those days, the wife had no say-so over her body.

Husbands were the first to receive the report of a pregnancy, and women could not have a tubal ligation without her husband's signature. My late spouse informed me that the results were positive. We selected an obstetrician so care could be started immediately.

The school term was almost over, so I decided to continue classes and complete the credits. In the meantime, we had started planning for the little one. We would convert our spare bedroom into a nursery. I was excited and told the family. Everyone expressed their joy.

Around the end of the first trimester, signs of fetal loss began to appear. A brief stay in the hospital was of no avail. All was lost. Tears followed for many years. When the same event occurred two years later, a barrage of testing was begun to see why the problem happened.

Various medications and procedures were attempted to no avail. The sight of moms cradling their babies was very painful for years. Mother's Day was a time in which I wanted to just disappear. All of the celebration left me miserable and uncomfortable.

With each client who lost her baby, I could truly empathize. I did extra studies and consulted various doctors to see in what way these moms could be helped to either conceive or retain their next fruit. Some were helped. Others had various conditions for which there was no help at that time.

Before in vitro fertilization became popular, there were just hopelessness and silent tears. IVF has solved some cases and brought happiness into homes that otherwise would have been childless. Only the childless woman who wants children understands another childless woman who wants children.

There are the moms who are dealing with premature and/or low-birth-weight babies. Premature babies and low-birth-weight babies are at risk for decreased survival rates. The good news about these births is that many can be helped. Moms who seek early prenatal care can help avoid these fates.

A program called Healthy Start was started in our state by one former Southern governor in the early 1990s. He had observed stress-related poor birth outcomes. He devised the program to help moms with the relief of stressors in their lives. Decreased stress has been shown to improve maternal outcomes.

Both Healthy Start and Healthy Families have been able to impact maternal outcomes through offering such resources as childbirth and Lamaze education and access to Medicaid, which provides financial assistance for prenatal care, labor, and delivery costs. Breast-feeding classes are also offered.

Women who are improperly nourished can produce undernourished and underweight babies that have other health problems. The WIC program (a feeding program) provides supplemental foods such as juices, milk, eggs, cheese, and formula. Food banks are accessible to the moms who are on the Healthy Start program.

There are many other programs included such as emergency shelter, child-care assistance programs, Job placement and training, help with GED and high school completion, and domestic violence referrals, to name a few. Clothing can be obtained at some of the church clothes closets.

As mentioned earlier, a program similar to Healthy Start is in service, called Healthy Families. This program works with the families longer. They provide family guidance for the family's children and connect families with programs that help to meet their needs. Moms with medical problems are mainly serviced by Healthy Start.

There is a section of Healthy Start called High Risk. This program hires more advanced nurses who possess more specialized skills. They follow moms who have more critical medical problems. They are usually stationed in the hospital, where they see these clients when they come into clinic for care. They also do home visits or delegate the visits to field nurses.

Clients enter the Healthy Start or Healthy Families program by way of referrals. They are screened for medical, social, financial, and other needs and problems at their first medical provider. They may be screened individually by a nurse or some other member of the health team.

Healthy Start clients are required to be screened, but they may voluntarily opt out if they do not wish to be followed by the program. They are required to be screened for problems on their first medical clinic visit. After their screening, they may also decline home visitation. The program is strictly voluntary.

The referrals are sent to a central office, where they are processed by clerical staff. The referrals are sent to the various Healthy Start and Healthy Families providers based on zip codes. The most acute and needy cases are usually found in the inner city.

Before strides were made in sanitation practices, maternal deaths from puerperal infection were not uncommon. Many women contracted the fever following an unsanitary delivery. Maternal fever at any stage signals the possibility of trouble to the health and well-being of both mother and baby.

While childbirth has become seemingly a relatively normal process, it is not without risks to both mother and baby. Moms should avail themselves to prenatal care as soon as they discover they will be producing new life. Early care can result in more positive birth outcomes.

Childbirth classes prepare the mothers for what to expect, which often allays their anxieties. The classes also include segments about care of the newborn. Boot Camp for New Dads is offered and is becoming more popular. It is a program that allows experienced dads to mentor new dads.

Some new moms are mentored by their friends who have given birth or by their experienced family members. Some clients informed me about the childbirth channel which they watched, and they found it to be helpful.

In any circumstance, knowledge and understanding about the birth process and surrounding events are valuable tools for all mothers-to-be. Informed clients seemed better equipped to cope with the birth experience.

When the women did not have housing, food, clothing, insurance, access to care, safety, and some sort of support system, this created more stress. Various agencies offering these services were mobilized and matched with clients needing the services.

There is a special section of Healthy Start which follows the babies after birth. The nurse who has followed the mom may be assigned to the baby or another nurse may follow the baby. The nurses collaborate on the care and decide what is best in the situation.

Multiple maternal and child health disciplines work together to assure that the mom moves through the system and obtains the services needed. The client is not dropped after delivery. She is given the opportunity to talk with and consult staff even after the case is closed.

Some clients go through the system with subsequent pregnancies. These ladies said they appreciated the home visits with all of the brochures and educational information provided. It also gave them the assurance that a medical person was in their home overseeing and helping where needed.

Postpartum is a most important phase of the delivery process that is often overlooked. Many moms do not return for their six-week check or postpartum visit. Moms need to be examined to make sure they are healing properly and there is no infection. Future birth plans also need to be addressed.

"Lo, Children are an heritage of the Lord: and the fruit of the womb is his reward. As arrows are in the hand of a mighty man; so are children of the youth. Happy is the man that hath his quiver full of them: they shall not be ashamed, but they shall speak with the enemies in the gate." Psalm 127:3-5.

Lack of children in Bible days was a source of shame and agony. Barren women were looked upon as outcasts in society. The birth of children, especially a male, was an important event because it meant that the family heritage would continue.

In biblical times, the first son was supposed to inherit the birthright. The birthright was a special blessing passed down from the father of the family. This blessing gave the first son an inheritance with certain rights, privileges, and authority over the family. He was the subject of great respect.

Several barren women of biblical times will be discussed in this work. Prayer was always the remedy for the barrenness during biblical times. I have seen several babies born to women who received prayer alone or prayer coupled with treatment.

While working in all areas where women were encountered, one fact stood out. If a woman could produce a child, she was accepted and inducted into the hall of womanhood. The one initiation standard was to be able to produce a baby.

Barrenness or infertility continues to be a problem with all of our modern-day technology. During my early nearing senior years, after elopement, my spouse, who was also advancing in age, wanted me to try in vitro fertilization. A longtime friend from a nearby out-of-town city, told me about a doctor who would do the procedure at any age.

I figured this was my last shot at motherhood before the biological clock quit ticking. Somehow the yearning for motherhood had not gone away, even at my age. The thought was exciting at first. After all, I had heard about a woman somewhere overseas that had given birth at age seventy, although I was not nearly that old.

I had heard about other births from women in their fifties and sixties. Why not me? Then the doctor told me I would have to obtain a donor egg from someone in my family due to my age. This was where I drew the line and decided it was time to give up my quest to become a mom.

Asking someone else for an egg seemed a bit much. I thought of all the legal and social implications involved. Having been separated from my family most of my life made it difficult for me to ask the ones I knew.

The thought of the exacerbation of any chronic illnesses in older women also deterred me from going through with the procedure. Suddenly I was faced with issues I did not want to address or go through with. Women with chronic illnesses have survived the process.

One of my coworkers confided in me that she had IVF, or in vitro fertilization, with both of her children. She stated she suffered from high blood pressure, was sick a lot, and had a difficult time. She said having two precious children was worth it. She was about fifteen years younger than I am.

Another coworker's daughter had birthed two children by way of IVF. She also had problems and miscarried twice. The procedure is fairly common but expensive. Some insurance companies will pay while others will not. I have known several other women who had the procedure.

Once and for all, I had to decide if all the trouble was worth it for me. I did not realize I was becoming more comfortable with the fact that childlessness perhaps that was to be my lot in life. We both wanted a child, but the weight of carrying, bearing, and rearing the child would be upon me.

Present-day problems did not seem to lend themselves to bringing a child into the world at our age, and abuse issues were present. Who would care for the child if we did not live to rear our child? Many children are already brought into the world with no consideration for their future.

Technology had come up with an excellent way to have the children I had so desperately wanted for years. Now my age stood in the way. This was my final opportunity to participate in Mother's Day functions and feel like I fit in. But somehow now, it did not matter. I felt secure in who I happen to be without meeting some quota or standard.

There are always foster kids and other kids needing adoptive parents. I had been reared by someone else who was not my biological mom. I am sure my foster mom would like to have had a child of her own. She did not have the choice, so she reared me perhaps as she would have reared her own.

The biological urge is stronger in some women than in others. It is underestimated and misunderstood. Many women weep silently over their barrenness while others hate the thought of having a child. Still others accept their barren state and move on in life.

For two decades, people had prophesied to me that I would have a child in my later years. I was regularly seeing special needs children being birthed by older moms. At my age, chances were very high for producing a special needs child. It occurred to me that I could not bear the thought of my child being ridiculed by cruel people.

Motherhood is an honorable status whether the child is one's biological, foster, or otherwise. What matters is that the child receives the love, care, and nurturing it deserves. Children respond to love no matter who gives it to them.

My spouse already had two adult sons and six grandchildren. He knew what it was like to be a dad. When we married at an older age, the furthest thing from my mind was having children. The idea sounded good at first, and it may have satisfied my lifelong urge to be a mom. At my age, it could have also been a disaster.

My love for children has made the work in this area a most enjoyable venture. The young moms have taught me much about life, the streets, and child rearing. Much of their advice and survival skills were never written in any textbook. I was supposed to be the teacher, but the moms taught me a lot.

All they needed was channeling of their energies, emotions, goals, and values. Many of them meet me in the streets today and remind me of my days with them. Many of them have gone on to make something of their lives. Some clients got married. Others went to College or bought homes.

Many of them redirected their energies into positive goals. Many times, we think our teachings and efforts go unnoticed. We go about our daily work and do not realize someone is looking for a role model. When they see it in someone they follow.

The ages of my clients ranged from thirteen to forty-eight. I encountered one nine-year-old who aborted early. The older moms said their pregnancies were accidental or they had a new young partner who wanted children. The bulk of the caseloads ranged from age sixteen through the twenties.

Mothers of many of the clients looked young and were very young themselves. They had wanted to spare their daughters from going through what many of them went through by having a baby at an early age. They had counseled and preached to their daughters to no avail.

Some moms put their daughters out of the home in their anger and frustration. Some of the daughters had to be placed in shelters and other facilities for unwed mothers. Many of the dads deserted the clients and would not support them during the pregnancy. Some dads disappeared for good.

Other women were in the city alone. Starry eyed, they came with a boyfriend, who then deserted them. Some came hoping to find a better life in the big city. Some of the clients came from nearby Colleges. They had been sent to College to learn, met some guy they thought loved them, and ended up with child.

In the Healthy Start program, strong emphasis was placed on recognizing and meeting the needs of these displaced women. Many times, the grandmothers needed to be counseled and calmed down. They could not imagine how their daughters could do this to them.

The Maternal and Child Health section would be incomplete without mentioning some of the women in biblical times that could not bear children. Infertility and barrenness are not modern-day phenomena. Childlessness in Bible days was a curse, as mentioned earlier.

The most widely known among barren women during biblical times perhaps was Sarah, the wife and half sister of Abraham. The story of Abraham and Sarah starts in Genesis 11:29-30. God had promised Abraham that he would give him a son.

Becoming the father of a son and a great nation was impossible with his present wife, Sarah. Sarah tried to make the prophecy come true. She sent her handmaiden, Hagar, in to Abraham to produce seed. Ishmael was born as a result.

When Abraham turned one hundred years of age, Isaac his son was birthed by Sarah Genesis 21:5. Sarah was ninety years old at the time of the birth Genesis 17:17. This birth was unusual with man, but not with God. "Is anything too hard for the Lord?" Genesis 18:8

A thorough study of the book of Genesis chapters 11 through 25 gives the complete account of the lives of Abraham, Sarah, and Isaac, the son of promise, and Hagar and Ishmael, the son of the bondwoman.

Another incidence of barrenness occurred in Genesis 25:21. Abraham's son Isaac's wife, Rebekah, was also barren. Isaac prayed for his wife to conceive. "And Isaac intreated the Lord for his wife, because she was barren: and the Lord was intreated of him, and Rebekah his wife conceived" Genesis 25:21.

Rebekah gave birth to twin sons. One of these two sons, Jacob, sired twelve sons that comprise the twelve tribes of Israel. One of Jacob's two wives, Rachel, was barren, but she later gave birth to two sons. "And when Rachel saw that she bare Jacob no children, Rachel envied her sister" Genesis 30:1.

Hannah was listed among the barren women. After being vexed by her husband's other fertile wife, Penninah, Hannah earnestly prayed to God for a son. She promised to lend him back to God. Because God honored her gift, he gave her five more children. See 1 Samuel 1:1-28, 2:21.

Another woman from 2 Kings Chapter 4 will be mentioned. This particular woman had befriended the prophet Elisha. She perceived that Elisha was a man of God. This prompted her to confer with her husband and make plans to graciously host this prophet whenever he came to her town.

This woman had great respect for the man of God. She wanted to do what she could to make his stay in their home as comfortable and enjoyable as possible. She had no idea that through her kindness, she would reap the benefits of having her own child.

She solicited the help of her husband to make the man of God's stay in their household pleasant. "As we have therefore opportunity, let us do good unto all men, especially unto them who are of the household of faith" Galatians 6:10.

"And it fell on a day, that Elisha passed to Shunem, where was a great woman; and she constrained him to eat bread. And so it was, that as oft as he passed by, he turned in thither to eat bread. And she said unto her husband, Behold now, I perceive that this is an holy man of God, which passeth by us continually" 2 Kings 4:8-9.

"Let us make a little chamber, I pray thee, on the wall; and let us set for him there a bed, and a table, and a stool, and a candlestick: and it shall be, when he cometh to us that he shall turn in thither" 2 Kings 4:10. This woman was simply being kind.

As a result of the woman's kindness, Elisha had his servant, Gehazi, to call the woman and inquire as to what he could do for her. Elisha was informed by his servant that the woman's husband was old and she had no children. Elijah prophesied to her that she would have a child.

Just as Elisha prophesied, the woman conceived and gave birth to a son. Elisha, being a man of God, was able to prophecy the future to the woman. The prophecy came true. One day when the son was older, the son died. Elisha prayed and God gave life to the woman's dead son again.

Several babies have been born in our church as a result of prayers by our pastor. Women who had miscarried many times or who had trouble conceiving came to the altar for prayer. Some parents who had babies have remained with the ministry while others have left.

Some of the moms had prayer along with medications and/or medical procedures. As stated earlier, at times, God uses medical science and the skills of the physicians for healing. At other times, he may supernaturally heal the person. God cannot be boxed in as to how he will accomplish something.

The mighty strongman Samson's mother was barren before conceiving him. "And there was a certain man of Zorah, of the family of the Danites, whose name was Manoah; and his wife was barren, and bare not" Judges 13:2. This was the famous Samson who gave the secret of his strength to Delilah.

"And the angel of the Lord appeared unto the woman, and said unto her, Behold now, thou art barren, and bearest not: but thou shall conceive, and bear a son. Now therefore beware, I pray thee, and drink not wine nor strong drink, and eat not any unclean thing" Judges 13:3-4

Samson's mother was given specific instructions as to how to guard her health and the health of her unborn child. Samson was to be an anointed child whose great strength lay in never having his hair cut. His mission was to deliver his people from the oppression of the Philistines.

Samson indeed delivered his people by slaying many of the Philistines. Unfortunately he divulged his secret of his great strength to a harlot who betrayed him. The Philistines blinded him and imprisoned him. He died with the Philistines while he was destroying them Judges 13-16.

The direct origin of the Philistines is a matter of speculation. They were considered as enemies of the Children of Israel. For further information about the Philistines consult *Smith's Bible Dictionary* by William Smith (pages 513-514). The publisher is Thomas Nelson.

The bringing forth of children into the earth is an awesome responsibility often taken too lightly. One only needs to pick up a newspaper or listen to the television to hear about the irresponsibility and problems connected with parenting these days.

Just as the enemy wanted to destroy Jesus, Moses, and all of the people that were used mightily of God, he is still trying to reach and destroy children. Many of these children are destined to be great in the earth. If the enemy can defile them before they are aware of their destiny, he will do so.

Parents need to pray for and with their children. Dads often are not aware of how powerful their prayers and presence are with their children. In cases where marriage is impossible for one reason or another, continue to pray for your children. Some dads father children while married to someone else.

I met one dad who fathered twenty-three children from different mothers. There was no hope of ever being a father to all of these children. Irresponsible parenting causes children to be shortchanged. He had to pay child support without a professional high-paying job.

Parents, beware of talking badly about one or the other of the child's parents. Something you say may cause the child to dislike his mother or father. That is biblically known as sowing discord among brethren. Children may grow up and hate you for turning them against the other parent, or other people, for that matter.

A number of such cases have been witnessed in my life. These parents wonder why the child hates them and have nothing to do with them years later.

They keep your grandkids away from you. You may be reaping the crop from the discord you have sown.

"These six things doth the Lord hate: yea, seven are an abomination unto him: a proud look, a lying tongue, and hands that shed innocent blood, a heart that deviseth wicked imaginations, feet that be swift in running to mischief, a false witness that speaketh lies, and he that soweth discord among brethren" Proverbs 6:16-19.

When seeds of discord are sown about a person, children don't know any better. They often believe the one who is giving them the most care and attention. This is a common practice with abusive spouses. They will tell the children a lot of untrue information to cause them to dislike the other parent.

Dads, don't deny your children now and then expect them to embrace you when you get old and need them. One Father's Day, I was playing for a church. A dad came in pitifully in tears. He talked about how he avoided his kids and refused them child support. He was now lonely, miserable, and rejected by his children.

Maternal, Child, and Dad health

The value of a dad in a child's life is immeasurable. So is having a mom. Man was originally intended to be the priest of the home and a helpmate to the mom. It is expected of him by God to guide his family in the way of righteousness. He is supposed to be the umbrella over his wife and children.

Some men take this to mean they are to beat their mates into submission. When a wise woman feels she is truly loved, respected, and wanted, she has no trouble submitting to the priest of the home. Some men are so far off track until they wouldn't know where to begin. Prayer is a good start.

Seeing a dad taking care of his children and spending time with them is a touching sight to behold. Seeing that positive self-esteem being imparted to the children ensures that these kids will be okay in the world of today. These kids are not likely to be among the negative statistics.

Being blessed with a biological dad and a foster dad gave me the advantage of seeing life from a protected point of view from both of them. I always felt safe even when I left home. Dads impart something that moms cannot.

There is an unspoken, masculine strength in good dads. Good dads make moms' work easier. Both of my dads started me out by filling me with biblical knowledge, which I still remember today. There are things they told me never to do, and today it is as if they are still saying, "Don't do that!"

Maternal nursing should be called maternal, child, and dad health. One of the most important components is left out. In olden days, when a baby was born, dads were sent out in the kitchen to boil water. The water wasn't needed. The midwife and everyone wanted dad to just get out of the way.

Dads are needed now more than ever to bring the family back into perspective and focus. There are times when dads go in the delivery room with moms and cut the newborn baby's cord. All dads cannot stand the sight of blood. They should be allowed back into the birth arena as soon as they can stand it.

While working Healthy Start, I saw a lot of the dads bond with their baby while it was still in utero. They talked to the baby, and many of the babies either kicked or showed some kind of response to the dad's voice. Even new babies seem to respond to a dad who has been present up until delivery time.

Premature babies who had the opportunity to hear mom and dad's voice often were the ones most likely to survive. The voice of authority from a dad does much to bring children into subjection. The fatherhood role can never be left out without something important being sacrificed.

Dads, you are needed. Get in there and provide that strength your mate and your children need. Don't jump in like a roaring lion; gently move in. You may not always be appreciated, but you are needed. Moms, help us out! Do your part. Show some love and respect where possible. Maternal, Child and Dad health refers to this concept of uniting the family.

Nursing the Incarcerated

The thought of a nursing job brings to mind hospitals or clinic work. As stated earlier, nurses work in many varied institutions and settings. Clients who are incarcerated are entitled to quality medical care. Local jails, state, federal, and prison rehabilitation institutions all hire nurses.

When we returned from the Western state experience, life ran seemingly smooth for a while. The secrets that were about to hit me in the face took about two years to surface. These secrets eventually destroyed our home and union. I did not know that the secret was that a love child had been created prior to our troubles and woes.

The situation of the love child could no longer be hidden, and everything came out in the open. Life went on as usual as these events unfolded. I had to work, so I took a local job with incarcerated children. This was an institution that housed what was known then as incorrigible children.

Cottage parents worked with the children around the clock for eight-hour shifts. Parents prepared meals and ran the cottages as biological parent would do. The children were required to keep their own rooms clean, attend campus classes, do their homework, and participate in recreational activities.

The children's stay at the institution lasted from one to two years, depending on their behavior. Each child was assigned to a counselor who worked with them during their time at the institution. When children had reached certain behavior goals, they were released back into their communities.

Recidivism was a problem for some of the children. Some of these ended up in a tougher program several miles away, and some of them ended up serving prison terms. Long-term studies are not known about the outcomes of all of the population that we served during that time.

Medical services will be addressed further in this publication. The program was pretty comprehensive in duplicating what was supposed to be a normal home life. There was a campus lockup. Lockup was reserved for children who committed infractions during their time at the school.

Kids who were caught smoking marijuana, fighting, breaking campus rules, or committing any inappropriate acts were relegated to lockup. When they had served the required amount of time, they had a hearing and were then released into the general population again. Their counseling continued.

Along with maternal and child health, my next choice of work was with children of all ages. Working with children often satisfies childless people's desire for children. Although all of us were children at one time, we sometimes forget what it was like being a child.

While working with children at any given age, I could see that their reactions to situations were no different from my own during my childhood. Children take their cues from adults and other kids as to how to behave. Example is a powerful tool in the eyes of a child.

A child who has been taken from an abusive environment and shown that there is a better way is likely to develop into a productive person. Watching children role-play often gives insight into what is happening in their lives. If they are being hurt, this comes out in their role-playing.

Working with youthful offenders was a most interesting field. A lot of the offenders did not have bad parents. There were parents who had done everything they knew to do in order to raise a proper child. Still other children had succumbed to peer and bullying influences to do wrong acts.

They had been coerced into doing some dumb act which landed them into the annals of law enforcement. Once they obtained an arrest record, regardless of their being a proper child, they were branded as a "bad seed." Children are faced with far more temptations today, which can be lethal.

Another class of children was those left alone with too much freedom and responsibility for their age. Unsupervised children do what they think is fun or interesting. A gun left unsecured looks like fun. After all, the people on television look like they are having fun with the guns.

One class of children that often got punished was the runaways. They got sent up for what I got away with twice as a child. Their running away was considered a crime. These runaway kids brought back memories of why I ran away. To any adult, running away is inexcusable and unacceptable.

All of us are taught either by example or by word about fair play. Children readily sense when fair play is not being practiced, especially if they have been taught otherwise. They cope with injustices as best they can. One reaction to perceived injustice or unfairness by children is running away.

My two childhood runaway escapades were followed by what I perceived as helplessness to the injustice that was either being done to me or was going to be done. The first is captured in my first book *Natural Bread Is Not Enough*. Fortunately, these occurred in a safer era of history.

Running away is often an act of cowardice, depending on what one is leaving. The child feels powerless to react or to show objection to the one who will mete out the punishment. As adults, we have more sophisticated ways of running away than the kids.

Adults run away by evading the bill collectors, outright lying, or moving away. There are other ways of evading situations. Fairness and fair play had been drilled into my head as far back as I could remember. Several things happened to me which I considered as unjust, so I solved them by leaving.

The first time I had been promised a trip to the county fair. Monies had been given to me, and more had been promised. Mother dear liked to dress me in coordinated colors. We could not find my matching light blue socks. They were later found under the bed. I was denied the trip.

The next runaway event occurred prior to the holidays after I got older. Mother dear had promised me no Christmas tree, no nuts, candy, or presents. We would spend the days before Christmas cleaning the house from top to bottom. I would be beaten if the work was not up to her specifications.

I could live with everything except the unreasonable beatings. I had done nothing to be beaten, and to just have to look forward to those horrible whippings was too much. A weapon of a large mulberry switch was displayed in plain sight as the threats went forth.

With a mixture of fear and resolve, I plotted a method to get away from this once and for all. I would not endure another beating. The beatings were becoming unbearable. I resolved once and for all that this injustice had to stop. Daddy B. and my foster mom's aunt seemingly were no longer offering little help with defusing MD's anger.

As the vacation time came closer and closer, my thoughts centered on the planned escape. I managed to keep my grade point average in the As and Bs. Homework was turned in as usual. I went about life with a mixture of fear and determination to end my perceived unjustified sufferings.

All of the other kids were excitedly talking about what their parents were giving them for Christmas. Every child looked forward to Christmas it seemed; I didn't. Even the poor kids could look forward to the goodies the churches and agencies gave them for Christmas.

As Christmas drew near, I reflected on the years of joy when we had a floor-to-ceiling Christmas tree. The heavily decorated and lighted tree stood on the screened-in front porch for all to see. The tree was always laden with presents and toys. Aunt E. took me gift shopping for family and friends' presents.

Our home smelled of pine fragrance throughout the holiday season. Christmas decorations and figurines were placed throughout the house. Poinsettias bloomed in the front and side yards every winter and Christmas. There were plenty of all sorts of nuts, candies, cakes, and pies during the season.

MD's aunt always brought out last year's rum-preserved fruitcakes. It seemed the pleasant Christmases were gone. I had been forced to stay up almost all night Christmas Eve of the past year. We cleaned the house from top to bottom, and I got fussed at all night about a stupid lost wig catalogue.

MD's aunt had also been a buffer for me. She had cushioned me from a lot of harsh discipline and hurts. She was getting older and becoming less effective at saying the right things to protect me from the onslaughts. MD had reprimanded her about interfering with her methods of discipline.

This is the reason nurses need to be trained to recognize subtle stress and abuse signs in children and young people. They also need to know what to do about it. Just because kids come in all seemingly well-behaved, looking good, and smelling good, does not mean all is well in their world.

Take opportunities to engage in conversation with children and parents. Much will be learned. I am not suggesting a witch hunt on parents, nor are all children being abused. I believe children will grow up feeling protected if they know the perpetrator's pain will stop at some point.

With the recent exposure of child harmers, knowledgeable, alert, and astute staff could make a difference in child safety. Impressive strides have been made recently in teaching children how to participate in their own safety. More surveillance and intervention wouldn't hurt.

Christmas vacation was drawing near. On the night before the last day of school, I collected a few clothes, shoes, and personal items. I carefully packed them in large brown paper bags and carried them out to the road behind our house. I would have had a problem if those bags had gotten stolen.

It never occurred to me either that the clothes could have been stolen or rained upon that night. When kids are desperate, they don't always make the wisest decisions. Sometimes they do downright stupid things. I sensed the wrong in what I was about to do, but I didn't know what else to do.

The writing is not intended to encourage kids to run away. There are far more dangers in the world today for unaccompanied kids than during my time as a child. Kids today are kidnapped, killed, tortured, and used as slaves. Safe havens exist for kids today, but not for those running away from home.

Finally, it was morning. I went through the usual ritual of getting cleaned up, getting dressed, and eating the last hot breakfast. Suddenly all the good parts of being here mattered no more. I am sure Christmas would have turned out okay, but I wasn't taking that chance. Enough was enough!

From the smug look on my foster mom's face, she knew nothing about my plans. She only knew she was about to have herself a great time beating up on me when school let out. I said, "Bye," and left. I quickly ran to the bus stop and recruited a few of my friends who helped me go to the road out back and get my bags.

They helped me get my bags on and off the bus and into my locker until school let out. Two of my sisters and one brother who had been bused to this school helped me get my things on the homebound bus. All they knew was that I was coming home with them for Christmas.

Ironically, no one queried me as to where I was going. My brother and sisters knew because I had told them. I did not tell them I was running away. I was afraid if I told anyone, I would go back to be flogged for the holidays. Any astute nurse engaging in conversation with me would have blown my cover.

Earlier, it was mentioned about the separation from my siblings. At first, we were all dispersed into different homes in different parts of the country. My maternal uncle who had these four siblings, eventually passed away. These siblings ended up with my maternal aunt. Their school started busing them to our school.

Another brother and a sister had been legally adopted into different homes in another state. The youngest sister died of accidental electrocution. She reached under a circulator heater to retrieve a dime. She was grounded on a wire. Precious time was lost in getting help for her.

Cardiopulmonary resuscitation was not common during that time. This sister died on the way to the nearest hospital about five miles away. Every medical person is required to learn and practice CPR now. I always encouraged my clients to become CPR literate, especially moms with small children.

Prior to this runaway day, I had met my siblings. As I was going to my hallway locker one day, I saw two girls and one guy who looked like the siblings I remembered. As we drew closer to each other, we recognized each other. What a reunion!

I informed this aunt as to why I ran away. I was afraid she would send me back to my Mother dear. *I would surely be killed and not see another Christmas*, I thought. After all, another mouth to feed during the holidays was not everyone's dream. My maternal aunt quickly made accommodations for me.

After we had spent a lovely evening of dinner and laughter, here came the big truck. This time, it was the same couple who had taken my older sister and me away from our parents several years ago. My aunt (who is now deceased) was not impressed with my foster mom's anger because she had a temper of her own. They had a brief verbal confrontation.

I heard Mother dear ask for me. I started trembling in my boots because I knew I was about to be sentenced back. I had not escaped the hard work and floggings after all. Then she said to me, "Give me back those clothes you took with you. When you come back, I will give them to you."

My aunt said, "She won't be back." I was left with only what I was wearing. This was a Friday, which gave my aunt time to pick up a few clothes from the rummage sale. We had less, but I was happy to be back with my family. The meanness and beatings ceased. I felt relieved and my prevailing feeling of stress left.

The truck finally pulled off without me, and I felt as if a ton of bricks had been lifted off my shoulders. After Christmas, I started working on Saturdays and after school. We wore some hand-me-downs, but they were clean and ironed. I was happy.

Living with my aunt and siblings was a great time of emotional healing. We often talked about our experiences with our foster and adoptive families. Five of us siblings were reunited in what was not the wealthiest of circumstances, but we were happy to be together. Our discussions about our experiences served as a debriefing for each of us.

As stated in another part of this writing, children do not like to be separated from their siblings. They also do not like it when their moms and dads separate. There is somewhat of a feeling of completion when all of the family is together. When that is broken, it causes stress to all involved.

For the first time in my life since being taken away, I could remember feeling relaxed and non-stressed. I no longer had the newest of clothes and shoes, but I went to bed every night with a full tummy. Having to get up early to be bused to the school was not an unpleasant experience because I was with my siblings.

Now I had to work to help myself with school expenses. Fifty to seventy-five cents an hour was a good salary for a teenager with no bills. I helped pay for some of the groceries, my school lunches, and supplies. I had been somewhat of a workhorse at my foster mom's house, so work was no problem.

Small salaries went a long way in those days because everything was cheap. I remember gasoline being seventeen cents a gallon in our small town. I even bought ribbons and socks for my younger sisters. None of the other siblings worked. My brother earned some funds playing the guitar and singing.

My foster mom had assured me that I would not leave her house not knowing how to support myself. She was right. I worked as a housemaid, babysitter, and a cook. I worked in the community cafe on Friday nights and some Saturday nights. There was always plenty of work for willing hands.

It seems everywhere I went people took me under their wings. The restaurant manager did so, and she taught me how to make the hamburgers, cheeseburgers, grilled cheeses, French fries, hot dogs, and over light as well as over well eggs. The manager allowed me to take leftover food from the day to my home.

The food from the restaurant helped to stretch food dollars at home. My siblings usually waited for me to get home, and we'd have a great time laughing, talking, and eating leftover restaurant food. I always had Sundays off work. We all went to church.

I had learned to play hymns back at my foster mom's church. I also learned to play by ear. I often sang in the church. When people learned that I could carry a tune on the piano, they called upon me to sing and play for various functions. That brought in small donations, which I greatly appreciated. My aunt bought a piano for me.

One summer, my aunt's daughter and her husband took me with them to work on two separate migrant camps. One camp was in Northern state and the other one was in state further up North. We lived in huts and shanties far away in the back woods. My cousin's husband had a truck, and he took us to work every day.

The migrant living situation was the pits. There were no indoor restrooms. Drinking and bath water were obtained from a yard pump. We got paid on weekends, at which time we went into town to buy groceries. My cousin's husband was one of the bosses.

It seemed people left from their hometowns to work the seasonal migrant camps. After that summer, I never wanted to go back. The same people went year after year. They never got rich although that was their dream. The idea was to save your money until you returned home. Work hours were 6:00 PM to 6:00 PM.

I learned to dig Irish potatoes from the soil, pick apples, and pick peanuts from the ground. We rode on a carrier behind a tractor. While on the tractor, we fed plants into a device that rolled them over and planted them in the ground. I resolved that I would never choose this as an occupation.

I could not wait for the school term to begin. The money was great for a teenager, but the work was the pits. My siblings were too smart to fall for coming on this trip. I was the adventurous one, and I really had an adventure! This would have been an ideal place to run a clinic.

Years later, when I became a nurse, I reflected back on the plight of the migrant workers. They lived in poverty and ignorance, waiting for the big payoff. They would become rich and never have to work again. None of them ever got rich. They had multiple social, health, and living problems.

When the men got paid, they got drunk on the weekends and resorted to fighting. People often got cut with pocketknives. They would bind up their wounds with a handkerchief, or they were taken to a medical facility in the city. No one ever died. Ironically, the police never came there.

Others went into the city to socialize in the local clubs and bars. I hated the fact that we could not go to church on Sundays. I was with people who were not devout in their religious beliefs. My cousins were the kind of people who occasionally dropped into church for weddings and funerals.

Finally, the day came when the migrant season ended. Everyone loaded into the trucks and headed for home. Some had drank and smoked up all of their earnings and had to borrow money to get back home. The migrant experience was a pathetic way of life. I had to avoid migrant life at all cost.

I was grateful that I had learned how to do an honest day of work besides this. Remaining in school was worth every moment. I was grateful for Mother dear's idea that a person should learn how to do more than one thing for a living. She taught me well.

We arrived home safely and not too soon for me. This experience left me with a greater passion for learning and greater compassion on the ignorant and unlearned. Unskilled labor was all most of these people knew. Some of them went on to work other camps when we returned home.

Upon returning home from the migrant experience, my siblings and I of course discussed it at length. It was a sort of debriefing for me. Much of my association with my siblings was a time of debriefing for all of us. Each one of us had lived through a lot of unpleasant situations and circumstances.

All of us had been beaten by keepers. It seems the homes that we went into had a lot of abusive adults. They were masterminds in thinking up punishments. As a public health nurse, many of the former foster youths told me they had abusive experiences in foster care. They learned to trust no one.

Many said they were beaten and fed the cheapest foods while their foster parents ate shrimp, crabs, steak, and lobster. One child said his foster mom made him suck the urine out of the sheets if he accidentally wet the bed. The proper authorities have investigated and corrected many of these abuses.

In one of my living communities, I transported a foster mom to her son's doctor's appointments weekly as I traveled to work. She told me I would be surprised at the number of foster parents who lived in our community. She said they fed the children hot dogs and peanut butter and jelly sandwiches.

These parents got by as cheaply as they could by purchasing the children's clothing from rummage sales and other outlet stores. Wherever the children went, they were easily identified as foster-care kids. They were poorly fed and they wore the worst-looking clothing.

Many of the teens who had graduated from the foster-care system did not know they had entitlements waiting for them. Some found out by accident. By the time others found out they had money, someone had already spent it. The money was allotted for the children's future lives.

Some of the children found themselves in institutions for youthful offenders following life in foster care. All foster parents have not been mean people. Some have been kind to the children and gave them a good start in life. Some still show the children much love and keep in touch with them.

One of my cousins kept foster kids for many years. No one could tell that these were not her biological kids. They ate the best food along with her and her husband. They were taken to the beauty and/or barber shop biweekly. They wore the best clothing and shoes from the better stores.

The children were reprimanded when needed, but never were they beaten. They were kept in school and taken to church on Sundays. When holidays came around, they were treated like family members. They were given nice toys and gifts. Most went from her home into adoption or back to their parents.

My former school friend, LT, also kept foster kids. The kids loved her because they said she treated them like a real mom. She too treated them as if they were her biological children. My cousin and my friend LT said their foster children still telephone them from time to time.

Nursing
THE YOUTHFUL OFFENDERS

All that I had gone through gave me insight into why many of these youths were committed to a youthful correctional facility. This was still the institution mentioned earlier. Most people did not want "bad kids" in their neighborhoods, so this institution was on the outskirts of town.

One girl said, "My parents gave me too much freedom and never whipped me. I wish they had, I would never be here today." Another girl said, "My dad, brother, and uncle molested me. I thought that was normal until I told my girlfriends. They ostracized me, and I got sent here after that."

Many of the youths said their parents had lots of booze and cigarettes lying around all the time. These vices were irresistible. Another girl had gotten into occult activities with her free time. She had a habit of running away from the school each time she was about to be released on good behavior.

The girl said she had gotten involved with a powerful cult and if she missed a gathering they would use her as the next victim. Many of them were involved in pot smoking, which was one of the strongest vices of our time. Cocaine use was rare.

Some drank excessively, while others were promiscuous. Among the population were an eight-year-old girl and her ten-year-old brother. They had killed their playmate and hid him in the bushes prior to being committed. They were never transitioned into the general population.

Here students were taught to release their anger in acceptable ways. They attended classes in the schools provided on campus, which kept them up with their grade level. Students were also taught social skills. They had a large community dance on Friday nights, where they could learn to dance and interact appropriately with other people.

There was a clinic which was run by us four registered nurses. We assisted the doctor with examining the youths on admission, clinic days, and sick call. Standing orders were used the rest of the time. There was some malingering occasionally. We used malingering time as health-teaching time.

Two nurses ran the day clinic while two ran the evening clinic until 11:00 PM. Children often came just to sit and talk about their particular issues and ask the nurses their questions. Just as teens are today, they were looking for answers they couldn't get from parents.

Every discipline of nursing was practiced in the facility. Health teaching was in great demand. Students were taught how to take care of their own bodies and how to avoid certain illnesses. They were taught how to prepare and eat healthy meals. Vices such as smoking and drinking were discouraged.

Awards programs were held periodically, where students were rewarded for good behavior or some accomplishment. There was a large campus swimming pool where students were taught how to swim.

The clinic was housed in a large bungalow-style building that had three sections. The clinic was situated in the front section of the building. The dental clinic was across the hall from the four-room medical clinic. Students received a medical assessment and a dental assessment upon admission.

Prior to the admission exam done by the pediatrician, the students were held in the intake portion in back of the building. The back of the building had its own entrance. Each student was screened from head to toe for illnesses, drugs, lice, body marks, scars, tattoos, and evidence of prior injuries.

Some of the kids were very resourceful at hiding drugs in their afro hairstyles, hems of their clothing, and in body orifices. The children, along with all of their possessions, were checked into the intake cottage. After a thorough bath, shampoo, and medical exam, they were held in the intake area until all tests and labs came back normal.

The middle of the building housed a four-bed area which was reserved as a sick bay. Students returning from the local hospital were held in the area and transitioned into the population as their condition improved. There was also an isolation area for hepatitis and other contagious illnesses.

Pregnant moms experiencing problems were also held in a part of the area until they were stable enough to be sent home to their parents. While the students were in the clinic inpatient area, we spent much time teaching them about their disease entities and how to take care of themselves.

All infections of any type were treated upon admission. We completed the urinalysis and the bacterial cultures in our own incubator. After completing venipuncture, we sent the specimen to a local lab for analysis. Immunizations were given if needed.

When all lab results were completed, each student was brought into clinic again. The pediatrician would go over the labs with the student. Any necessary treatments were prescribed at that time. We dispensed the necessary medications from the clinic.

Students, along with their house parents, were taught what medications they were being given. They were told what side effects to expect and to report to the nurse. The five rights of giving medication were practiced. These are: the right medication, to the right patient, via the right route, the right dose or amount, at the right time.

Students had the liberty to discuss their condition with the nurses at all times and to ask any questions they had. We were always open, honest, and candid with the students. They loved it, which kept the lines of communication open between us and them.

A long-term love child situation came to full circle in my home life. I learned of this, and it brought about conflict and marital dissolution. My life changed drastically again, and I moved from the area. I returned to the Western state to live with a relative. I needed to sort out my life and future direction.

While in another city out West, I lived with my cousin who operated a home for psychiatric clients. Her business was in her own home. I assisted her with the clients by administering whatever care they needed, such as cooking for them and administering their medications. She kept five clients.

Some of the clients were on lithium shots, which they received at the psychiatrist's office periodically. My cousin was a strong positive caregiver. The clients were all well managed. She took me and them, my six-year-old twin cousins and another eight-year-old cousin swimming every morning.

She had an organized and well-rounded day for the clients and us. My cousin took us sightseeing sometimes, and she had another cousin to take us to see the town at other times. We had family gatherings and cookouts almost every night, which she conducted in her very large home.

After about a year with my cousin, I decided to return to Florida. I was not getting a salary for what I was doing, and I felt like I needed to restart my life. We discussed staying in staying out West versus going back to my home down South. Someone had convinced me that the West had some potential disasters worse than the storms of the South. I went home.

Upon returning to the South, I was in need of a job. I had not preapplied prior to coming home. When I returned home, I applied for two nursing jobs and one job at a popular shoe store. The shoe store would have meant immediate employment until a nursing job became available.

The shoe company called me right away, but fortunately the nursing job had called first. Ironically, in a night vision, I had dreamed of myself working in a glassed-in facility. At first I thought it was the local hospital to which I had applied because it had a glassed-in nursing station.

Sometimes we overlook dreams and visions, but sometimes they are trying to show or tell us something. If one is indwelled with the Holy Spirit, He leads, guides, directs, and shows us information for our good. The vision was a supernatural occurrence that showed me specifically where I would be working.

My present pastor often warns against always looking for manifestations versus making sure our dreams and visions line up with the word of God. We are to rely on God's word when it comes to dealing with manifestations. We need to be grounded in God's word.

The supervisor of a prison rehabilitation institution called me for an interview. The interview was successful, and I was hired on the spot. Sure enough, the entryway and the nursing area were totally glassed in, as I had seen in the vision.

The job fell in place like clockwork. I started to work within days of being hired. I was soon able to get an apartment and get my life back on track. I started playing for revivals and other functions in the area. Work was productive and pleasant despite being risky.

Nurses rotated shifts around the clock, with eight-hour shifts per nurse. I mainly worked nights and evenings so I could be available to play for Sunday morning services. My life began to come back into perspective and focus. I continued my life of playing and singing in revivals when I was off work.

Triage and assessing complaints were also a large part of our job. We worked closely with the medical staff to provide comprehensive care to all residents of the facility. The inmates always adopted a protective attitude toward the nurses. The inmates encouraged each other to respect us.

For example, if one of the males used profanity or spoke disrespectfully in our company, the others would verbally reprimand him. There was an amicable group of workers during my tenure at the prison rehab. This seemed to transfer on to the inmates so that we coexisted peacefully.

These men were being trained to return to society as productive citizens and givers instead of takers. They had the option to learn various trades, which many of them did. The prison guards were well trained and acted in a way as to command respect. The residents very were focused, it seemed.

Nurses were required to make medication rounds to each building every four to six hours and prn. Prn meant medications were given as needed. Clients were observed and assessed for any aberrations in health or levels of consciousness during medication rounds.

A prison guard accompanied us as we went on our medication rounds. Clients were locked in cells, so we had to be given access by the building guards. Inasmuch as all of the clients were goal and education oriented, few seemed interested in committing acts that would get them kicked out.

Occasionally clients who were let out for recreation would start a fight. Bruises would result, necessitating that the nurse carry first aid supplies along with the medications. Staff had to be alert to avoid carelessly leaving items around that could be crafted into a weapon.

After spending time in forensic nursing, I started getting the desire to move on into an area where I could work with children. I moved to a larger city where there were more opportunities to practice pediatric nursing. I was offered a job immediately. I came aboard after notifying my previous job.

The large teaching hospital had children of all ages. The pediatrics department ran the gamut from nursery clients to eighteen-year-old clients. I worked nursery and pediatrics for two years. I was satisfied to spend the rest of my career here or to get into public health.

The temptation of a much higher salary offer in the cardiac care unit across the street drew me in. Training was free, and there were much better benefits. This hospital eventually moved to another section of town. Since I wanted to remain where I was, I applied for and got into public health.

The prison rehabilitation program appeared to be a great idea to me. Residents are often released from prison with no current job skills. While they spent time behind bars, society moved along without them. Upon returning home, they discover that they have no way to carve out a life. Recidivism is likely.

Most employers will not hire them, thus they have no way to earn income. With no legitimate income, nothing else happens for them. I am no expert in these matters, but it seems rehabilitation would be far more cost effective in the long run. Being taught a marketable trade seems reasonable.

According to a Florida Department of Health survey in January of 2012, it cost $53.35 to maintain one prisoner per day. Annually that computes to $19,473 per person. While working with many of the inner-city women in one town, I encountered some who were convicted felons.

Some of the women had served time in some penal institution. As a result, they were barred from many opportunities that others take for granted. They could not access HUD (housing and urban development), jobs, or College. Trades were also closed to them.

Every avenue to success they tried turned out to be a blind alley. Several of the women were very academically brilliant. They had unfortunately made the wrong decisions at an early age, which ruined their chances at pursuing a successful career. Parole officers can sometimes help them.

The boot camp programs and the police athletic association programs, such as PAL, have good ideas to avert behaviors that eventually lead to a life of incarceration. We may not be able to offer much to the ones who are already in trouble, but we, as nurses, can encourage moms to involve their wayward kids in the available helping programs.

Community counseling programs also exist. They may be found in the phone directory. Presently in a lot of cities, there is a local help line number that activates access to other help lines. Most cities have a network of helping services which can be fairly easily accessed.

One twenty-five-year-old inner-city mother of seven told me she had started her life of crime when her mother kicked her out of their apartment. She was kicked out because she refused to allow bodily favors to the mother's boyfriend. She and her sister were later placed into the foster-care system.

The client said she and her sister ended up in a series of abusive foster homes. They acquired a history of running away and eventually started stealing food from stores just to survive. Eventually they were caught, jailed, and since—by then she was eighteen years old—she served time as a convicted felon.

She, as well as other clients, made money by pole dancing, bootlegging, hair braiding, and selling whatever they could. This particular lady was very industrious, academically endowed, and could have succeeded at anything she attempted. She was able to do quite well for one so disadvantaged.

PUBLIC HEALTH

After working several years in various hospital roles, I got the opportunity to work in public health. Public health was my first choice of nursing work, but the low staff turnover in the town where I lived kept all nursing positions filled. I accepted a public health job after three more years of nursing.

My first assignment was with the North West clinic. Although there was a central health department downtown, there were many satellite clinics strategically placed throughout the county which assured access to every resident of the vicinity.

The North West clinic was located in a heavily populated, inner-city area of town. The clinics were filled every day. Various clinics also ran concurrently some days. The primary health clinic serviced adults with acute and chronic illnesses. Each clinic had its own laboratory and medication room.

A licensed practical nurse was hired to draw blood and complete the lab requisitions, but we all, at one time or another, had to assume the position as the lab person. Our supervisor believed in cross-training everyone. We also did pregnancy testing and immunizations.

Well-baby clinics were held at different times during the week. Babies were brought in at intervals for well-baby assessments and shots. The babies were seen by a pediatrician or by a nurse. Ill babies were treated by the doctor.

Ill babies were treated and medicated as needed. Educational information about the child's condition and treatment was given by the nurse, either verbally or written. Mass Medicaid screening clinics were held periodically mainly for children who were on the Medicaid program.

Children were screened and treated for lead poisoning, vermin, head lice, and other problems. Various stations were set up for each entity to be tested. Children were weighed in and screened for vital signs, vision, hearing, and blood pressure.

All were sent to the lab for urine testing for diabetes, infection, or any abnormality. When all testing was completed, each child saw the doctor. Appropriate immunizations were given, and parents received copies of their children's tests. Blood work was done where applicable.

Referrals were made if children needed to be seen by other disciplines such as the psychologist, surgeon, further hearing and vision screenings, or anything beyond the scope of the clinic. Nurses completed any preventive educational instructions.

Family planning clinics were also held in the building. Women received annual medical testing before being given birth control. Pregnancy testing was also done prior to giving birth control methods. Clients were also tested and treated for infections and any other illnesses.

After three years in the clinics, a new population of clients began to be seen at that time. These babies screamed a lot and were seemingly inconsolable. Astute doctors and nurses discovered that these babies had been exposed to illegal substances such as marijuana and crack cocaine.

Programs for testing the moms and babies at the time of delivery revealed that moms had used substances during the pregnancy. Many of the affected babies were removed from their mother's custody. Some went into foster care. Others went to aunts, grandmothers, and other family members.

Moms realized their babies would be taken if they tested positive. Many of them went across state lines to have their babies where there was no testing. They returned after a time with their babies. The babies eventually showed up somewhere in the system due to other health problems.

One of the nursing supervisors formed a nursing team to visit and provide nursing services to these babies. I was given the opportunity to work with these families and their babies. We were required to attend various trainings to learn how to take care of these babies and their moms.

We were required to provide the caregivers with methods to console these babies, such as swathing. With the screaming tendency, these babies were at risk for abuse. Premature babies are also at risk for abuse. These babies were irritable and did not fit the usual sweet and cuddly baby mold.

Grandmothers and other caregivers did wonders with these babies. They possessed the patience and caring skills these babies needed. We followed the babies as they grew into the toddler and elementary school level. Some of the babies later showed hyperactivity and learner disability behavior.

Some were very smart. When I returned from my Broward County Health Department experience, I visited a couple of the homes to see what became of the babies. I was surprised to find one six-year-old very much into Christianity. This male was aspiring for the ministry and preaching.

Another child whose grandmother was a minister and prophetess was also doing quite well. She had taken charge of most of his rearing. She allowed his mom to take a lot of the responsibility for his care. He was bathed in love and prayer by his grandmother.

Four years later, I began contemplating a move to the Ft. Lauderdale area. My older brother, oldest sister, and other family were living in the area. I had been communicating with my brother, and I decided to try moving. After applying for a transfer and getting the job, I went down to the area.

I decided to work and complete the move gradually. I owned a condominium and could not leave immediately. I had to sell, so I traveled until I could make permanent arrangements. Selling was not easy because condominiums were inexpensive and not widely desired. Association dues deterred a lot of sales.

PUBLIC HEALTH IN SOUTH FLORIDA

Two years of my public health nursing were spent in a South Florida clinic. Near the end of my studies for the master's degree in Theology, I put my Bible College studies on hold and went ahead with a transfer and a partial relocation.

Upon successful transfer to the health clinic down South, I went to work without a break in service. It was a good feeling being around my family again. I lived with my brother with the intention of selling everything at home and purchasing a home down there.

It was my intention to link with a South Florida Bible College as soon as I got settled. I put my condominium up for sale and commuted biweekly to and from home to the Southern area. At that time, apartment condominiums were very plentiful and difficult to sell.

Association dues deterred buyers. Assessments can increase at any time. The difference between apartment living and condo living is that you purchase your unit, the association affords some protection, the grounds are kept, and there are laundry and swimming pool facilities. Mortgage liquidation is possible, but the association dues continue forever.

Living upstairs limits yard space. Condominiums are ideal for retired people who want to lead a simple, fairly protected life. When owners sell their units, these units often become rental property. Neighbors become transient, which is not always a plus.

My few potential buyers wanted the property on a rent-to-own basis or off-the-record sales for little or nothing. Neither method sounded kosher, so I decided to keep the place. Traveling to check on the property biweekly was fine for a while. In the meantime, buying a home in South Florida became a possibility.

Homes with zero to five hundred dollars down payment were in drug-infested neighborhoods. People had moved away to get away from the crime. I decided to remain with my brother a while longer. We lived in harmony and fun, and we spent a lot of time reminiscing about our lives.

My nephew and I spent our time attending just about every function there was around town. We saw every movie there was at that time and ate tons of popcorn. My nephew taught me computer skills and how to play video games.

He taught me about the library system in South Florida, so I eventually resumed my Bible College studies by correspondence. After watching the class videos, I mailed in the homework for my grades. I visited the home campus periodically to do my speaking requirements.

True to form, I found a church to play for in the area and resumed my piano playing. Holidays became fun again as I spent them with my family. Time flew while I was down South, as I enjoyed the days with my family.

Upon arriving at the South Florida health clinic, I was taken to personnel to complete paperwork. I was given the grand tour of all the clinics and introduced to all of the staff. These were some of the friendliest, most congenial people I had met in a long time.

All staff was comprised of just about all nationalities. I worked with a lot of Hispanics, Haitians, Jamaicans, and people from other countries. The clientele was just as varied. I was placed in charge of clinics immediately. The work pace was much more brisk than from where I left. I quickly adapted.

Staff workers from other countries were very diligent. They completed tasks so quickly until I had trouble giving them enough work. All workers were focused, and everyone cooperated with duties until all assignments were completed. Everyone was very respectful of authority.

My salary almost doubled because of the area. I also received a cost-of-living raise and hazardous pay because of certain dangers associated with home visitation. When I received my biweekly pay check, I thought someone had made a mistake.

Personnel in the human resources office assured me that this was what I should be earning. Annual raises came automatically. The high income allowed me to be able to help my family and to maintain my own affairs back home. There was even money left over for savings and other desires.

Clinics were overcrowded. I'd never seen so many people coming for services. They came by appointment. Others were seen in what was known as a triage clinic. Every day, an assigned clinic nurse was given the task of treating the triage population and deciding who should stay and see the doctor.

The clinic from which I came was very large, but I had never seen so many varied problems, illnesses, and needs concentrated in one place as this health clinic. This was a job as well as a mission's field. A nurse could spend her days meeting needs within as well as outside of nursing.

People in charge could easily pass over the problems of the clients or put them off. Clients could be turned away at triage or accommodated at the nurse's discretion. Inasmuch as many clients were from other countries and were not accustomed to the American system, many of them were unaware of what they were entitled to have.

Many of the foreigners spoke little to no English. They brought their children to interpret. Others used our nurses from their native lands to interpret for them. Some were illiterate and required much help with navigating the system. Had it not been for the cooperative and cohesive staff, working here could have been a real challenge.

Out of all the hordes of people, clinics went surprisingly smooth. Camaraderie held us together like glue in accomplishing every task. The clients were also very grateful to us for helping them. None of the clients ever showed any disrespect or displeasure for the services we rendered.

The decorum and discipline of the children in the South Florida clinics amazed me, except on one occasion. The children sat quietly and orderly beside their parents. They talked only in a soft tone of voice. I had seen this type of well-behaved children in Israel, the Netherlands, the Bahamas Islands, and Canada.

One of the families in the South Florida clinic had brought their children for services. Ordinarily the kids were well disciplined and quiet. For some unknown reason, this particular little boy decided to test his dad's limits. His dad verbally reprimanded him strongly, but he ignored his dad.

The child continued to run about and be disruptive. Dad had that "Wait until I get you out of here" expression on his face. Dad managed to contain himself; Mom watched in silence as if she also knew what was coming. The family made it through the clinic visit, and then they left.

Several days later, the same family came back for a follow-up visit. The child that had been disruptive remained quiet and well behaved beside his parents and siblings. We all suspected that dad's discipline had made a little angel out of that kid. There were no scars or signs of abuse on the child.

A generation of babies was also being exposed to crack cocaine during my stay at the clinic. Moms were on the streets while relatives took responsibility for the babies and children. Babies who were born with withdrawal symptoms tested positive for cocaine.

One day, a very distraught grandmother brought five grandchildren to clinic. Grandmother said her daughter was on cocaine and on the streets, so she took the children to keep them from going into the system. It appeared as though these kids had pretty well worn their grandmother to a frazzle.

These children had very high energy levels and were in perpetual motion. It did not help that the grandmother was very soft-spoken. She needed shot records brought up to date and transferred to immunization forms, school physicals, and all of the workup that went with them

This was a day I could have easily told the grandmother we can't get the records or she would have to reschedule some of the children. As I looked on that weary, beaten-down grandmother, a wave of compassion passed over me, and I could not deny her requests and needs. Everything got completed.

By the time the grandmom left our clinic, her entire countenance had changed. She was smiling and expressed how encouraged she was that all of this paperwork was completed and she could get the children in school. Her needs consumed a great deal of clinic time, but it was worth it to see her smile.

During my second year at the health clinic, I was unanimously elected nurse of the year. This was the highest honor a nurse could receive, and I will always be grateful to my former colleagues. All of the physicians were kind, considerate, and personable.

In this clinic system, we were required to rotate through all clinics. The main clinics consisted of well baby, sick baby, maternity, pediatrics, primary adult care, immunizations, and triage. Other clinics included family planning, epidemiology, and infectious diseases. WIC was also housed in the building.

Evening clinics were held in order to accommodate working clients. All of the clinics were housed under one roof in one large building. There were other similar clinics situated throughout the county. The evening family-planning clinics were mainly staffed with MDs, nurse practitioners, RNs, and techs.

A pharmacy was also housed in the building. This made it easy to be sure clients got their medications, birth control methods, and clear instructions before leaving the building. A laboratory was also included in the building, so lab results were readily available to the doctors.

Time was drawing near for me to return home. I was feeling the pinch of the thirteen-hundred-mile-per-month commute. I had been tailed by other automobiles a few times on I-95. During an early morning commute, a car came out of the median strip and followed me.

I kept driving until a big rig rounded the corner. I got on his tail and flew with him into the next large county. Upon reaching the larger county, I was able to lose the person in the heavy traffic. God took care of me. I knew it was time to cease commuting and return to my residence.

During that time, being younger than I am now enabled me to commute without it wearing me out. The biggest problem with commuting to me was that it consumed so much time on the road. One deacon from the Southern church said to me, "Sister, a rolling stone gathers no moss."

He was saying I would never acquire anything in life as long as I drove that distance monthly. I already owned a furnished condominium and a new car. I was a tither and a giver, so it wasn't as if I had not accomplished anything in life. I lacked nothing at that time.

Not being able to sell my condominium and feeling the leading of the Holy Spirit to return to Bible College was what finally made me return to my home. I reconnected with the local health department. God caused some blessed things to come my way almost as soon as I came home.

The job was threatening to lay people off and withhold paychecks. The doctor in charge of my workstation called me in his office and asked if I still wanted to work. I said yes. He wielded his authority, and I never lost a day's work or a paycheck. God assured me of work.

I was allowed to keep most of the raises I had received while working in the Southern area. Only the hazardous pay was taken away. I was able to return to the area of my choice when I returned to the home clinic. I also received the county health employee of the month award that year.

The last day of work finally arrived. All of my Southern clinic coworkers expressed their joy of having worked with me. They gave me the feeling that they truly did not want me to leave. I felt wanted, needed, and loved by staff and family, yet I knew I had to return to my home.

The royal red carpet of goodbye was rolled out. Some of the best cooks had brought out some of the most scrumptious dishes for the festivities. Everything was well prepared. Many of the staff members gave me money and many lovely gifts.

Someone gave me an address book, and everyone put their names and addresses in the book. We still remain in touch until this day. Unfortunately I never got a chance to see the director of nursing again, as she passed away soon after I left. She was a true jewel during her lifetime.

I left with a new respect for people from the Southern clinics as well as those from other countries. When a friendship is developed with them, it is a true one that can only be broken by you. As with other areas, this area that I was leaving had its own brand of good folks and hospitality.

Abandoned children, disadvantaged people, and those who have experienced unusual hardships in life tend to sense insincerity more readily than those who have been sheltered all of their lives. A disadvantaged single mom who has had to fight her way through life can spot insincerity miles away.

Many of the single moms in the Southern clinics and the Northern clinics intuitively know how staff feel about them. One valuable lesson to learn early in nursing is to be as sincere as possible with clients or choose an area where you do not have to directly encounter people.

Develop positive bedside manner and home visiting decorum. Watch what you say in front of and to clients. If you are angry or short-tempered, do not try taking it out on clients. Never be condescending with clients, as they are also people with feelings. Their being ill does not make them inferior to us as professional workers.

All medical institutions have a system of reporting staff members who are out of order. Clients are often reluctant to report staff members who mistreat them. Many are afraid of retaliation of some sort. Others have shared to me that they hate to see the person lose their job.

"Be not forgetful to entertain strangers: for thereby some have entertained angels unawares" Hebrews 13:2. This is mentioned to stress the importance of positive client contact. First impressions do indeed tend to be lasting. I have heard clients say of some staff: "There's that old mean lady again."

The lady may have been very nice, but she allowed her bad day to get in the way of her contact with people. We all have our days when we'd rather not encounter anyone. Life's necessities often require that we encounter each other. Make it as pleasant as possible.

Public Health—
The Return Home

I returned to my home town clinic. The relocation did not happen. I missed my family, but I knew I had things to accomplish at home. I reconnected with the Bible College and completed the requirements for the master's degree in Christian counseling.

While attending evening classes at the Bible College, I worked days at the clinics. During the Wednesday night Bible College classes, each student was required to prepare and deliver a sermon from the current class's information. I resumed my classes and the music scholarship with the College.

Public health is thought to be offered only for the poor. Public health is for all people. Public health touches all areas of our lives whether we know it or not. A few of the departments units and their functions will be mentioned in the upcoming pages.

The clinics are only a segment of this giant operation. The Bureau of Vital Statistics is a part of the health department, and it involves everyone born in the state. Birth certificates and death certificates are processed and issued by this department.

Epidemiology assures the safety of food at restaurants and eateries. Public eating places must adhere to certain regulations. When food-borne illnesses occur, the source is tracked by this department. An investigation is launched, the source of the offense is visited, and the problem is resolved.

Communicable disease outbreaks are also investigated and handled by the epidemiology department. Such diseases as hepatitis, measles, West Nile virus, influenza, encephalitis, and other diseases must be investigated for their origin. Nurses visit clients who are affected for case finding and teaching.

Water testing is done within the health department to assure that the public is getting safe water. Periodically, we hear of boil water alerts. These are handled by the health department. Swimming pools must be regulated for safe water. This is handled from the health department.

There is a chronic disease prevention program that addresses diabetes, smoking cessation, cardiovascular health, breast cancer, and other such disorders. Surveillance and treatment are continuous for AIDS, tuberculosis, and socially transmitted diseases. Contacts are visited and serviced.

The lead program conducts continuous work to ensure that children and adults are free of lead poisoning. I encountered two children who had lead poisoning. The department and I worked together to see that these children received chelation therapy.

When children live in old houses with peeling paint, they may be exposed to lead. The paint is usually lead-based. This lead can cause brain damage in children. Children sometimes peel the paint and eat it because it has a sweet taste. Lead poisoning can cause death.

A very large and most important department unit is emergency preparedness. This department orchestrates activities and programs to ensure public safety during hurricanes and other catastrophic events. They keep the public informed by working with the media as well as officials on a local, state, and national level.

Since the events of 9/11, this department has enhanced its efforts to keep health department employees in a state of preparedness to respond to any and all events as needed. Mock disasters are staged periodically, where employees and officials can update and renew their disaster skills and responses.

Emergency preparedness works with Homeland Security and FEMA (this is the acronym for Federal Emergency Management Agency), when dealing with disasters. An incident command system goes into operation and takes whatever measures necessary to carry out public safety plans.

A feeding program called WIC which is an acronym for "women, infants, and children" has been a part of the health department for years. It helps to supplement babies with formula. Prenatal clients and new moms, as well as children up to age five years can receive WIC services.

A breast-feeding program is included in the WIC program. Recently, we worked with a family from one of the Samoan countries. Healthy Start assigned me to help this mom. Mom was having problems with breast-feeding. By collaborating with WIC, we were able to help her.

The family had not activated WIC because they spoke little English and did not understand American customs. They were not familiar with what else to feed the baby because breast-feeding was their means of feeding their babies. Mom was distraught. The baby was apparently frantic from hunger.

I had prearranged a call to the health department's language interpretations department on my cell phone. The lactation nurse and I made a home visit. The lactation nurse was able to talk the mom through the process by way of the interpreter on the cell phone.

The baby's grandmother, grandfather, dad, and aunt were present in the home. The whole family had just migrated to our area, and the dad was the only one employed. It was not quite time for him to go to work. When the mom successfully fed the baby, the whole family rejoiced.

They invited us to sit down and have something to drink to celebrate this great accomplishment. We all drank WIC Juicy Juice fruit beverages and rejoiced. Subsequent follow-up visits revealed that the breast-feeding efforts had been successful and the baby was gaining weight.

Dental services for children up to age eighteen are offered through the health department's dental clinic. There is also a mobile unit called the Happy Tooth Express/ Smile Express that goes about the city servicing children. Adult clinics are also available through the public health system.

School health is also a part of the health department. Nurses assess the health status of school children and provide services as needed. Each nurse is assigned to one or more particular schools in the county. Children at special-needs schools are also serviced.

School health nurses are very instrumental in collaborating with clinic nurses and Healthy Start nurses to provide more comprehensive services to schoolchildren. They make sure school physicals and immunizations are current. They assess and service sick students as needed.

The interdisciplinary team approach assures comprehensive coverage of the entire scope of clients' needs. Referrals are activated where necessary to complete the services. If clients plan to relocate, they may be referred to or connected with services at their intended destinations.

Some clients have been connected with neighboring county health departments, WIC, and Medicaid. They were assured continuity of care. Clients have also been known to have their information transferred to other states, thus avoiding costly duplication of services.

Many of the obstetrical clinics issue their clients a booklet known as a passport. This passport includes information about the client's prenatal status. It is brought to clinic and updated during each visit. If the client moves or delivers at another hospital, she has her information with her.

Environmental health helps to ensure the safety of such businesses as tanning salons and body piercing salons. Sanitation of the environment is one of their main functions. Their work is multifaceted. They intervene where toxic elements are present in the environment.

Many of the disciplines within the health department have what is known as field service. Employees conduct home and field visits depending on the nature of the problems. Field staff visit homes to provide surveillance, education, and care as necessary.

Substance abuse impacts a large part of almost every community. Nurses and social workers provide services through the health department's substance abuse program. They conduct home visits and provide care and referrals as needed. Some attend court sessions with clients.

Substance abuse staff visit and collaborate with the correctional and rehabilitative staff in jails and various centers throughout the city. Affected mothers and babies are visited at home, and in the institutions as necessary, for the purpose of providing care and education.

A multiplicity of departments and services are always functioning in the health department concurrently. They are vigilantly working at all times for the health and safety of the community. Nurses work in practically all of these areas. Health departments are located in most cities.

Working in the public health department offers the feeling of working many types of jobs all at one time. Various units within the department offer a different type of work. Variety abounds. Home public health appealed to me because people are in a more natural environment.

Hospitals serve their purpose of caring for clients with acute illnesses. There are more community emergency clinics now, and many problems can be resolved without entering a hospital. While hospitals are very necessary, some clients try to avoid going there.

Having been out in the community a lot has allowed me to see clients who would rather suffer through some illness than to go to a hospital. They do not want to have to deal with the household disruption that goes along with hospitalization. When care can safely be done at home, it should be.

Men particularly hate the thought of hospitalization and going to a doctor. When a medical person comes around, they get a lot of their questions answered. Many have been encouraged to seek further medical care to prevent further damage to their bodies.

One large problem encountered during my public health days was people with high blood pressure. They were avoiding medical treatment. Many were taking home remedies such as aloe juice, vinegar, or garlic. They were encouraged to at least keep up with their pressure at their local fire station.

They were given information about the consequences of untreated, long-standing high blood pressure. Some eventually started treatment while others decided to stick with their remedies. One man said he wants to leave this world all in one chunk . . . not piece by piece.

He meant he did not want anything removed or tampered with. His friends complained of impotence with the blood pressure medication, and he would rather enjoy life and then die. People tended to be more relaxed and candid in their home environments when discussing medical issues.

Home visitation has changed over the years. Medical people and nurses were highly welcomed in the home in the past. If you're known, you are still pretty much accepted. Home invasions and thefts of babies and children have rendered people more cautious of strangers showing up at their doors.

Some clients confided that they were afraid someone was showing up to either take their children or to stop their entitlements. It is not an unjust act to try and give the client a phone call before showing up at their door. When uniforms were worn, clients reacted more positively to visitors.

Others took special care to make their homes clean, nice, and pleasant when they knew the nurse was coming. Some put bows in their little girls' hair and did special things to make the nurse feel welcome. Some would offer their WIC Juicy Juice or a glass of cold water as refreshment.

Public health nurses were once identified by their navy suits or navy dresses. Some wore the blue public health beret or cap. Pinstriped light-blue cotton suits or dresses once identified public health nurses. Public health nurses carried a special bag similar to the doctor's bag. Name tags were worn.

The public health bag usually contained oral and rectal thermometers, blood pressure equipment, gloves, measuring tapes, and other supplies for assessing the mom and baby. Baby scales and adult scales are often carried along now, in addition to the above items.

Teaching materials are taken into the home, depending on what needs to be taught. An audio-video player is sometimes taken into the home for enhanced teaching. The health department's childbirth educator especially teaches a lot by way of the player.

Some local hospitals now have their own childbirth education programs. These programs are often held in the evenings or at night. New moms learn what to expect from the childbirth process. They are given a tour of the hospital and the delivery suite.

The moms are taught the Lamaze method of childbirth and how to breathe to relieve the discomfort associated with childbirth. Moms are encouraged to bring a partner to assist them in becoming familiar with the events that will take place at birth. Partners can also serve as coaches and helpers.

Some of the classes include breast-feeding instructions and care of the newborn baby. Moms who availed themselves to the classes have said they felt more comfortable about caring for their babies when they went home from the hospital.

An advantage of visiting the moms after birth is that they are given the opportunity to talk about the experience and obtain closure. They can also show the nurse what they have learned about cord care, circumcision care, bathing, shampooing, and generally caring for their baby.

The mom is given the opportunity to express her fears and ask for help in areas in which she feels uncomfortable. Time is focused on mom's diet and care of her own needs, which may sometimes be neglected while caring for her baby. Moms are also observed and helped if postpartum depression seems to be a factor.

There have been moms who were in town with no family or significant other. Some depended on friends, while others were referred and connected with support groups. The Healthy Families program does wonders with these clients. Healthy Families can work with the mom and baby up to five years.

While hospitals and inpatient facilities will perhaps always exist for the acute clients, public health is a popular health alternative. Outpatient surgical units, wound care units, and community emergency walk-in clinics are replacing the long waiting times once seen in hospitals and emergency rooms.

DISASTER NURSING

Nurses are trained and expected to function in disasters and emergencies. Prior to the hurricane season, health department nurses and other personnel undergo weeks of training and preparation while still carrying on their daily assignments. Special training has also been required since 9/11.

An incident command system remains permanently in place for all disasters. Calling trees are set up, and employees are drilled as to which employee they will be expected to call. Other calling systems are set into place, and employees are expected to be abreast of developments. They must also be available to deploy.

Each employee is assigned a shelter to work during the hurricane event. There are shelters designated for the general population and special-needs shelters set up for the infirmed, disabled, and aged. Patient placement is determined by triage, the client's living area, and a pre-registration system.

An emergency operations department is in place at all times within the health department. Other disasters and mass destructive events are planned for, whether they happen or not. All health department employees comprise one of the front lines from which disaster workers are deployed.

A sudden catastrophic event in one's life can be called a disaster. It can be on a local, personal, or massive level. It can cause great harm physically or mentally. Inner reserves can see us through along with community agencies' help.

Floridians and coastal residents deal with the annual dreaded hurricane seasons. Fire storms have also occurred and created disasters. Disasters that leave people injured or homeless are the most devastating. Deaths also often occur which affects families and significant others adversely.

For coastal residents, the hurricane season starts June first and extends through November thirtieth annually. Meteorologists track the paths of the season's hurricanes and tropical storms through the designated time. Coastal residents faithfully observe the forecasts in order to be ready to evacuate if it becomes necessary.

One such disaster occurred during the hurricane season on August twenty fourth, of nineteen ninety two. The infamous Andrew blew into the South Florida area with a fist of iron. One city's water tower was all that was left standing. The area looked as if it had been hit by a bomb.

Nine months earlier, I had moved from the area. Although mainly areas of South Florida were devastated, the city in which I had lived sustained considerable damage. Rooftops were blown off, trees were toppled, and power lines were downed. Other areas sustained damage from flooding.

Volunteers were recruited from within our health clinic. I served two separate deployments. The combined skills from working hospitals and community health were invaluable assets to my success as a disaster nurse. All nursing trainees should beef up their disaster skills.

When we received our assignments to report to the disaster area, we boarded a special bus that took us directly to our hotel during the first deployment. We were given dinner in the hotel's dining room. We enjoyed a good night's rest, which would be the last such rest for a while.

The next morning, we reported into the command center for our instructions and assignments. We were joined by other South Florida nurses and agencies. We were given information about what happened, where we were to go, and what we were supposed to do.

We were accountable to our supervisors. We were divided up into teams and were given designated areas to work. Assignments were alternated so no one got burned out from one particular assignment. At times, we worked as clinic nurses in the makeshift tent clinics.

At other times, we went from house to house to assess the status and the health of the population involved. We determined who had untreated injuries, who needed immunizations or tetanus shots, and who needed to be transported to the hospitals.

Some people had been without food and water for three days before anyone could get into the area to help them. By the time we got there, food, water, clothing, and supplies were pouring in from around the USA. As stated in my first book, people stood in lines for hours to receive basic necessities.

Tent cities were beginning to be set up as housing for the people. Many of the homes we visited had areas blown off such as walls, windows, and parts of the roof. Everywhere we went, people told us horror stories of how they survived. The one prevailing survival strategy was prayer and togetherness.

One family said they ran from room to room to survive falling debris. Each room they huddled in started collapsing. They would go to another room, and that room would start to collapse. Finally, they all crouched in the bathroom. That was the only room that did not sustain damage.

Some survivors said there was an eerie redness to the sky and a deadly calm just before the devastation hit. People who waited until the last minute to go to a shelter started out but did not make it. They were killed by debris and/or fallen power lines. Some were killed in their own homes.

The purpose of all of the planning and warning of the public is ultimately for everyone's safety. Many people try to ride out the disaster, which is never wise. Every person should keep all of the necessary storm supplies recommended by the hurricane center.

Prior to the hurricane season, the media increases its public awareness campaigns about storm preparation and survival. Newspapers print sections of hurricane editions with evacuation routes. People are advised to storm proof their properties and to stock up on their hurricane supplies.

WAS THIS A BOMB BLAST OR A HURRICANE AFTERMATH?

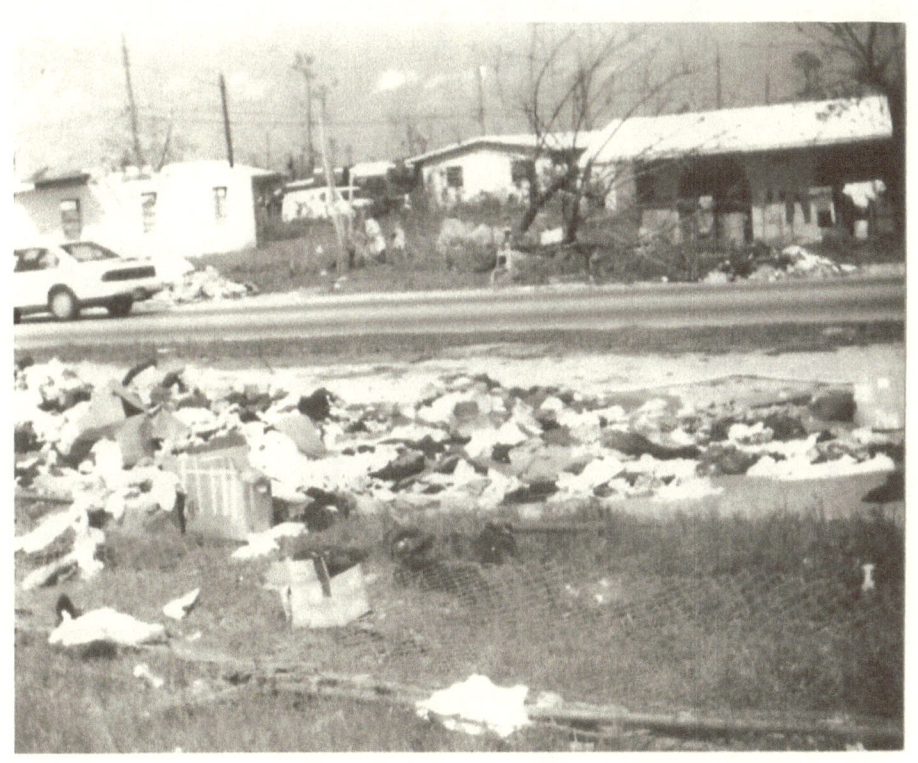

Our local team posed for a photo

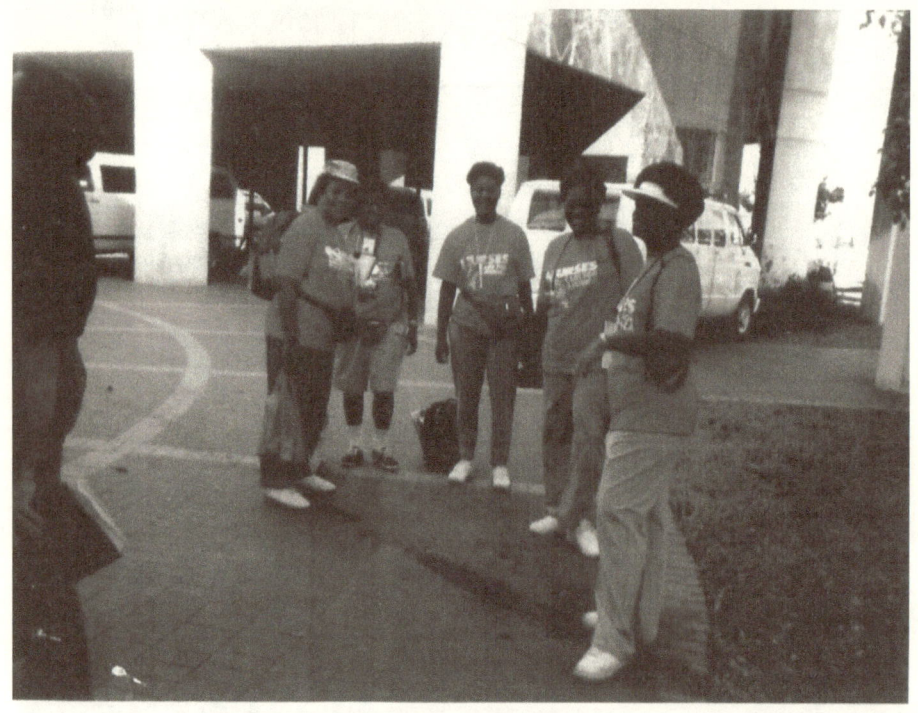

Our local team posed along with our military team

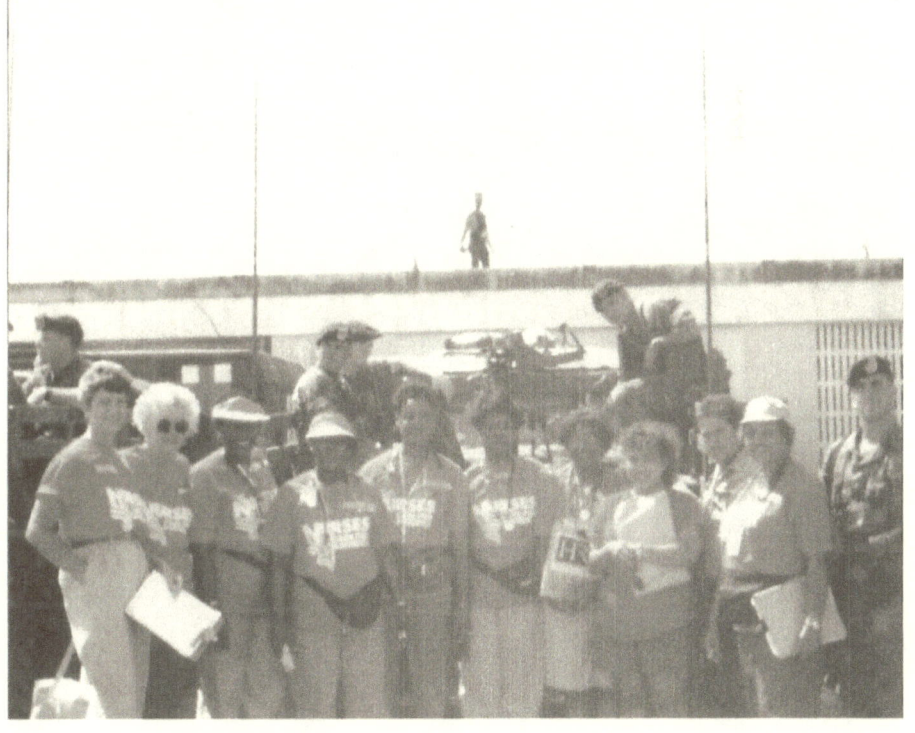

Million-dollar mansions were destroyed

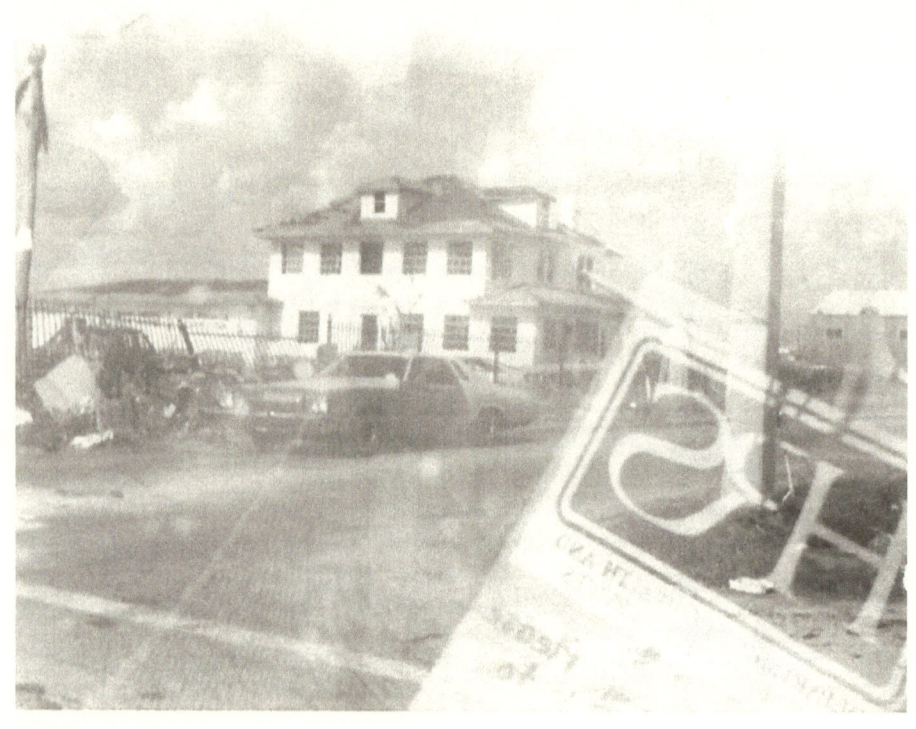

Our second deployment to the hurricane was a little more in the rough. We lived in a tent across from the makeshift tent city clinic. All of the other hurricane survivors also lived in tents. We had outdoor toilets only, and we had our own community shower. It was somewhat humbling.

Early rising was part of the plan. We had to get a shower and get to the makeshift food tent for breakfast. We ate army rations and then reported for duty. We worked in the tent city clinic all day and into the night. There was a never-ending stream of people with problems and medical needs.

We worked until everyone was serviced. We relieved each other for lunch, dinner, and breaks. There were times when we worked into the night such as when a mom went into labor. Assisting the mom until she could get to the hospital was one of our duties. One mom even named her baby after the hurricane.

When we finally went to bed, we had to sleep under mosquito nets to keep from being eaten alive by the mosquitoes. One client jokingly said, "These mosquitoes are so large, you can't swat them. You have to punch them out." We had no luxuries and no air conditioning. It was a true camper's delight.

One of the advantages of public health nursing is the freedom to work independently and to follow the doctors' standing orders. Much of the time, we were given standing orders. Doctors were freed up to attend to other matters.

We were able to work and blend harmoniously with other social and medical disciplines such as the Red Cross, social workers, law enforcement, and the military. The tent city operated somewhat like an ordinary city. All agencies worked together to try and help people put their lives back together.

People acted as though they were very grateful for everything we did for them. No acts of kindness by us seemed to go unnoticed. Clients verbally expressed their gratitude to us as they came and went from the clinic. We returned home feeling as if we had made a difference in the world.

Other hurricanes have followed for coastal and the surrounding areas. But no recent hurricanes have been as devastating to this area as that one. Other disasters such as the fire storms have occurred. People were displaced, and their lives were changed forever.

Reading various accounts of the Mississippi hurricane it seems to have been much worse than the one we experienced. When people are involved in disasters, one cannot make a judgment as to which disaster was worse. All disasters change lives forever.

Prayer, preparedness, a spirit of volunteerism and education continue to be our most potent defenses against the force of nature known as hurricanes. Organized emergency management and warning systems are indispensable to all cities and municipalities in emergency situations.

Our clinic resembled the tents that were set up for various services for the victims. People needed help in getting back on their feet. Homeowners needed ways to reach their insurance companies. People had other business issues that needed to be addressed through the social services.

Although we worked out of a tent, it was set up like an ordinary clinic. We had the usual supplies found in a clinic or an emergency room. When necessary, we had the resources and staff on hand to transfer clients to area hospitals. Some procedures went beyond the capabilities of our clinic.

A lot of people had to be immunized for prevention of tetanus. There were many people who had abrasions, cuts, and bruises. Some people did not have documentation of their latest tetanus shot. When one's tetanus shot was nonexistent or last date unknown, they were reimmunized.

Children who had no evidence of ever being immunized had to be reimmunized. Moms are encouraged to always keep up with their children's records so as to avoid unnecessary immunizations during a disaster. If you relocate, always take a copy of your child's shot record with you.

Following a disaster, especially storms and flooding, waterborne diseases can easily and quickly spread among the population. Mosquitoes can proliferate just as in Miami. They can spread some diseases such as the West Nile virus, Eastern equine encephalitis, and malaria.

With lack of adequate refrigeration during a disaster, food-borne bacteria can cause sickness and/or death. Flies also become a problem if there is relaxed technique in handling food and waste. Sanitation and careful hand washing must be practiced.

Prior to the days of immunizations, many people especially children died of preventable diseases. Smallpox was one of the first diseases for which a vaccine was discovered. A nurse came to our school and administered our first smallpox shots. Many of us still bear the smallpox scar.

Children need not die from smallpox, diphtheria, tetanus, whooping cough, polio, measles, mumps, rubella, pneumonia, flu, hepatitis, or any of the preventable communicable diseases. Many free immunization programs exist throughout the country in health departments.

Despite free immunization programs, many parents opt out of getting their children immunized for one reason or another. When an outbreak occurs, un-immunized children are at greater risk of dying from the diseases than the immunized children.

As we went through the neighborhoods of the devastated areas after the storm, we immunized many people who had not come into the clinic. The area had not yet been cleaned by city crews. Strewn glass, nails, and debris were on the ground. Everyone we met was compliant with the immunization program.

The water tower stood as the only witness to the existence
of one city after Hurricane, of August 24, 1992.

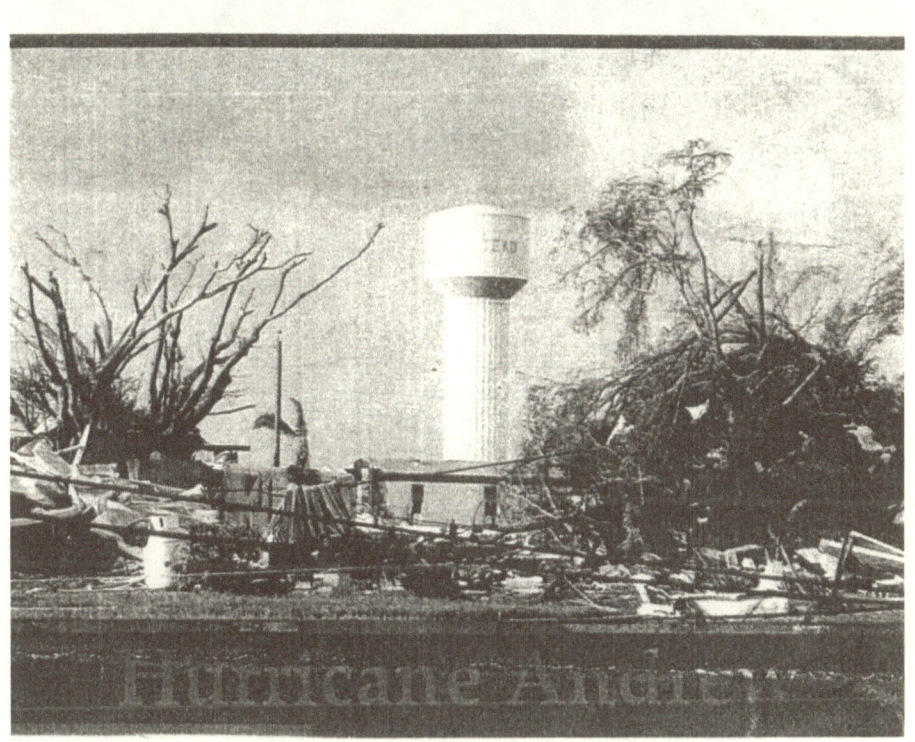

Tents, such as the one below, served as stations for social agencies, our clinic, our temporary housing, and the clients' housing

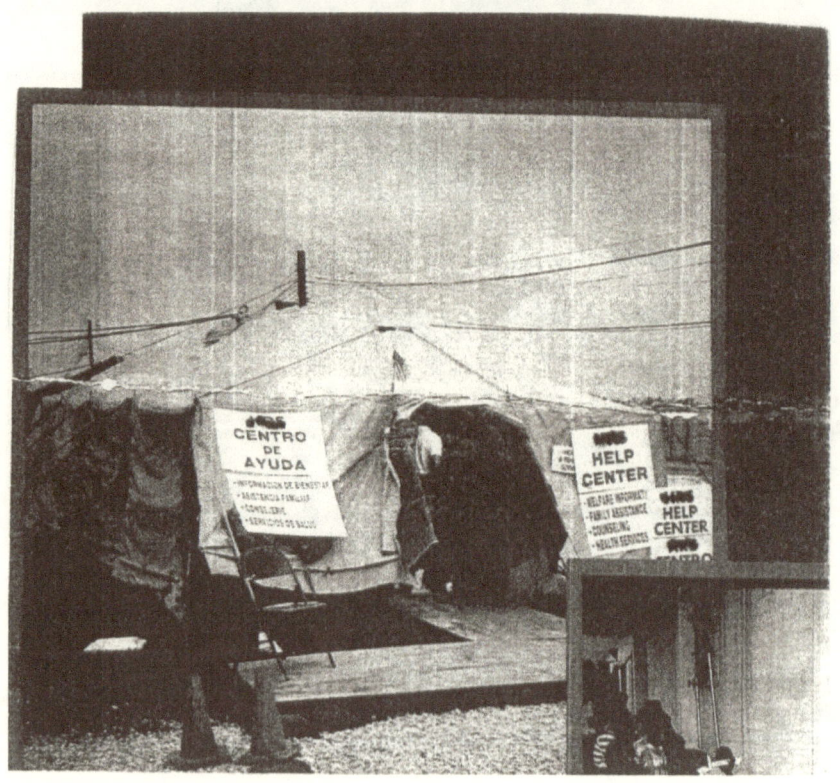

As we boarded the buses to return to our nice, comfortable homes, we felt blessed that we had been spared a blow such as the one we had just witnessed. The entire experience was humbling. Sleeping in a tent under a mosquito net was no fun compared to a comfortable air-conditioned bedroom.

A new appreciation for creature comforts came into my life at that time. If I had to choose between residing in the Andrew aftermath versus the migrant camp, I perhaps may have chosen the migrant camp. At least we had a solid roof over our heads, sleeping bunks, and no mosquito problems.

In the Andrew disaster, people had no choice. Brokenness in their lives was a fact. I saw much thankfulness among the local residents. There may have been some complaints, but I never heard one. Everyone showed gratitude. We never appreciate what we have until it is gone.

I have heard many people say we should live every day as if it were our last. We should treat people as if it were our last encounter with them. In the course of everyday business, those sayings may not be easy to live up to. We should try.

While visiting in the post storm area recently, there was no hint of the past devastation I witnessed with the storm. People had rebuilt and survived. They had pulled their lives back together. Knowing that God supplies inner resiliency gives us the determination to rebuild and move on.

Compassion also took on a new meaning for me. As I worked with the public health clients who lacked resources; it caused me to work a little harder to access available resources for them. What we discard and take for granted, other people would be very grateful to have.

To anyone contemplating a nursing career, public health is the place to see how some people really live. Everyone was not poor. While some may have been poor, others lived comfortably. There are times when staff members look down on clients and remark, "They can do better than that." They snicker at people's run-over shoes. What happens to another can always happen to you.

I have seen instances where purchasing food over a bar of soap was the priority. The advent of food banks has been a blessing. I have encountered people Dumpster diving, and it was not just for fun. It was their way of trying to obtain a meal. What would they give for a full belly of fresh food?

When I ran away from my foster parents' comfortable plush home, it was hard at times not to think about the creature comforts and the pretty clothes I left behind. While I was happy with my family, it would have been nice to have both family and nicer things.

Working kept me from being hungry. Trying to reach educational goals kept me busy. Singing and playing music kept me preoccupied and reasonably happy. Living in lowly surroundings, and not having much, kept me humble. Praying and reading the Bible kept me encouraged.

HOME HEALTH
AND AGENCY NURSING

In recent years, as hospital costs began to spiral upward, nursing began to return to home and community health on a greater scale. Hospital stays shortened, but people still needed care beyond the usual hospitalization period. In years gone by, home health was common.

Clients often feel better when they can recuperate in their home with family and friends. Home health gives the clients more freedom to resume some home activities. They do not have to lie in bed in a hospital wondering what is going on at their residence.

Medical personnel come in as guests, render their particular services, and then they leave. The client has the say-so of what happens in his home. Medical personnel are guests in the home, and we need to respect the home as such.

Before the Hospice was an established service, people chose to be brought home so they could be with loved ones in their departing hours. People often fear death and do not want to be alone when it occurs.

In other cases, people do not want a death to occur in the home for various reasons. This is where Hospice comes in. During my elementary school years, it was not uncommon to have the deceased relative displayed in the living room. This occurred with a family member of one of my teachers.

The person was a young child who had developed leukemia and passed away. We were taken to the home to view the body. We were fearful of the dead. Adults transferred their fears and superstitions of the dead to us, and we wanted no part of death in any home.

We like to think of home-health clients as candidates for getting well and eventually leading normal lives again. This is often the case. In other cases, the clients may be elderly, disabled, or they may need long-term care. Long-term-care clients are often sent to other community nursing facilities.

I have spent many years visiting maternal clients and their children as opposed to the medical clients. This type of nursing has provided a wonderful opportunity to foster positive health habits. It has provided a means of teaching clients to prevent illnesses before they occur.

It has also provided a means to assess needs in the home so these needs could be met by other disciplines. A mom may have needed help with groceries or her utility bills. Referrals were made to the appropriate agencies, and the help was provided.

As medical costs spiral, home health will perhaps be far more in demand as well as an option. In a recent home-health-care situation, the client was severely bodily disabled but was very mentally sharp and alert. The person was able to conduct business on the phone in his own home.

Home-health nursing has been a source of moonlighting for me at times. The first time, I was sent to work in a prison on the outskirts of town. This was a job on Friday and Saturday nights, 7:00 PM until 7:00 AM. This was one of the most hostile places of my entire career.

Nurses had to go into the crowded cafeteria to administer evening medications. Some of the belligerent clients would try to make remarks to provoke an argument or a confrontation with either staff or other inmates. The atmosphere was charged with anger.

Female clients had to be awakened and brought to clinic in a single file for 3:00 AM medications. As some of the women came up to the medication window they would spit at the nurse. I'm sure I would be angry also if someone awakened me at 3:00 AM for medications every morning.

After working with friendly clients most of my career, this was a challenge. I soon decided moonlighting was not for me and I would just have to manage with less money. The other nurse who encouraged me to join her at this job soon quit. We both decided moonlighting wasn't for either of us.

Ironically, the clients seemed to do well with the staff that treated them roughly and talked to them in coarse language. The louder staff yelled at them, the more compliant they became. I was baffled to the point of wondering why someone would prefer rough treatment over kindness.

The guys back at the rehabilitation prison were so different. They were more humane. If they uttered any profanities, they apologized to the nurses. I wondered what could have happened to so many of these women and men that could have made practically all of them so hostile.

This is one of those instances where I had to back off and apply my own medicine. This is one of those times when the phrase "Physician, heal yourself" applied. I silently prayed for those young people. Many of them appeared to be in their early twenties to fifties. Some good destiny had been aborted in their lives.

When children are born into the earth and they are anointed for some great destiny, they are targeted by the enemy to be destroyed. If they are not kept constantly in prayer by someone else, their lives will eventually be destroyed. All of us need the continuous light of the word and prayer.

Reflect upon the number of great criminals in history and how quick minded they were. Bonnie and Clyde would have made a great evangelistic team. Their wiles would have benefited many had they used them for good. They were deceived into thinking their crimes would benefit themselves.

This part of agency nursing would definitely be left to other workers. My job in this case was to make this a new prayer project. After all, we are commanded by the word to visit the ones who are sick and in prison. "When saw we thee sick or in prison, and came unto thee?" Matthew 25:39

Aging and End of Life

While discussing issues on the passage of time with a family member, we reflected on the subject of our older relatives. We both noticed that very few of them were left. We asked ourselves, "Where are all of the old people?" We came to the conclusion that we are the old people.

We both had exceeded the half-century mark, and we were so clearly reminded that none of us came on this earth to stay. No matter how much money we amass, how much property we acquire, and how much power we think we have, we will do as King David said, "Go the way of all the earth."

"Now the days of David drew nigh that he should die; and he charged Solomon his son, saying, 'I go the way of all the earth: be thou strong therefore, and shew thyself a man; and keep the charge of the Lord thy God, to walk in his ways, to keep his statutes, and his commandments" 1 Kings 2:1-3.

In the preceding chapter, David continued to admonish his son, Solomon, because he wanted to see him become a great king. David had been a great king, and as he was about to enter into eternity, he wanted his legacy of godliness to continue. He expressed his death as "going the way of all the earth."

All of geriatrics is not a time to be morbid and spend one's days focusing on death. It is not to be ignored because it is nearer than ever, neither is it to be dwelled on because there is still breath and potential. Continue to embrace life with enthusiasm.

Old age has been a very productive time for some notable people: How many people did eighty-one year old Clara Peller impact with her gruff, gravelly voice in the Wendy's commercial, "Where's the beef?" While people took notice of the hamburger, they also laughed and were amused by her candidness.

Anna Mary Robertson was an American folk artist known as Grandma Moses. She lived from 1860-1961. History is filled with productive elderly people. Productivity is one of the assets that inspire long life. When we cease to dream and look forward to the future, we cease to live.

As stated in my earlier book, the cemetery is filled with unwritten poetry, unwritten songs, and regrets from those who failed to fulfill their inner dreams. Many people tell me, "I really want to write a book one day." Others say, "I always wanted to learn to play the piano."

Just make your arrangements and get started! One of my university professors who taught the geriatrics classes always told us, "You're never too old to start anything you really want to do." Many elderly people have ventured into high school and College and completed their goals.

When younger people see older people accomplishing what seems like the impossible, they become inspired and say, "If they can do it, so can I." Even if you cease to live in the middle of what you started, at least you gave it your best shot. Life is not about us. It is about who we helped in our sphere of time.

"A good man leaveth an inheritance to his children's children: and the wealth of the sinner is laid up for the just" Proverbs 13:22. While we spend a lot of time acquiring possessions in this life, we need to acquire with the idea of who we can bless while we are here and after we are gone.

God did not intend for us to sacrifice everything in our lives for everyone else at all times. He wants us to enjoy some. Neither does he want us to be selfish and never help others. He said, "I am come that they might have life, and that they might have it more abundantly" John 10:10.

Many of the patriarchs such as Abraham, David, and Solomon, his son, were very rich. They enjoyed the wealth God gave them. They used their wealth to bless their families, strangers, their progeny, and themselves. While we may not be as rich as our patriarchs, we can take an example from them.

A sister who recently visited me was appalled that I was living in a humble condominium as opposed to a palatial dwelling with millions of dollars in the bank. What she did not know is that I could have had all of that had I not chosen to be generous and giving all of my working adult days.

As we age, we think about wills and who we will want to enjoy our possessions after we are gone. Often what is precious to us doesn't amount to a hill of beans to an offspring. Parents often will houses and lands to children who see no value in them and lose them to taxes.

At other times, children inherit money, and pretty soon they have run through it and are broke. Recently, a relative inherited a home and property from her adoptive parents. She had lived in apartments and other substandard housing for years. When her parents died, they left her a nice house with a nice yard in which her children could play.

The relative and her husband occupied the house for a while. The husband was killed in an auto accident, and the relative eventually lost the house. The mortgage had been paid off for years. The relative did not pay the taxes, and the city now owns the property.

When Daddy B. passed away, Mother dear called me and sat down with me. She told me she knew she was not going to live forever, and she wanted me to go through the house and get any and everything I wanted. She said, "The freezer (large chest model) is full. The freezer and its contents are yours."

She spared nothing and offered me everything they had acquired over the years, including the orange grove across the street. She said, "I want you to have anything you want while I am alive to give it to you." She also willed me and her favorite nephew three bank accounts.

Somewhere between the lawyer and the executrix, the money got away. We never got it. They turned out to be the parents I wish I had treated with love, patience, kindness, and tolerance over the years. Treat everyone kindly. You never know who will help you when it counts most.

As a whole, growing old in America is a very unpopular thing to do. Jokes about old people are cracked on television and everywhere else. Companies start mailing out offers for hearing aids, special insurance plans, burial plans, hum-around motor scooters, and all kinds of appliances.

Free dinners and financial planning seminars abound for the elderly. While all of these serve good purposes, most people can find what they need and want. Unfortunately, many of us neglect our health for years, which makes a lot of these items necessary.

One's genetic makeup plays a great part in what happens to our bodies as we age. Time on the earth also affects our bodies. Some people live to reach one hundred-plus years, while others barely make it to the senior years. Longevity is an asset, especially when health remains good.

Poor health and longevity can result in a miserable and boring existence. Without regular activity, exercise, and a proper diet, our bodies become less-efficient machines. Mobility may decline which limits ability to go whenever and wherever we desire.

The world becomes a smaller place to the elderly who cannot remain mobile. If there is no one to assist the elderly in getting around, many are confined to wheelchairs and walkers. The lack of speed in getting around sentences the person to life in a smaller world.

Many elderly people retain their mental sharpness. This makes them think they can accomplish the same activities they did in their younger years. Some find themselves accident prone because their mental function did not decline with their body's ability to get around.

While the senior years serve as comedy fodder for many, some organizations have made provisions for the comfort and respect of those of declining years.

Names will not be mentioned here, but these organizations have done much to preserve the dignity of aging.

There was a time when medical people referred to the elderly as "Grandpa," "Auntie," "Baby, "Sweetie," and such names. Current teaching is that people of all ages should be respected and addressed by their name. If the name is not known, look for it in their record or ask the person.

Our English teacher taught us many years ago that people who use terms such as "Sweetie," "Honey," and "Baby," when addressing any person are ignorant. Some people don't care what they are called, and others become highly offended by the names.

There should really be no such thing as growing old gracefully, since all who live long enough will grow old. Looking one's best is not the wrong thing to do. Make the best of it by contributing as much good as possible to society. Leave a legacy of some sort to family, friends, and/or strangers.

The problems of the elderly are real and undeniable. Problems such as diminished eyesight and loss of teeth result in the need for eyeglasses and dentures. The magnifying glass is often a necessary tool. Hearing may diminish, especially if the person has been exposed to loud noises for many years.

Bladder and bowel functions may be affected, resulting in the wearing of padded plastic underwear or a catheter. The problems vary, depending on the health of the individual. Some elderly are in excellent health and do not appear to be their stated age.

Whatever the status of the elderly, they need to be respected for their contributions whether large, small, or nonexistent. Grandma or Grandpa may have seen the family through many storms and crises. They should not be thrown into the corner as old rubbish.

Daddy B. was confined to a wheelchair prior to his death. He was very masculine, independent, and could not abide the idea of being waited on hand and foot by anyone. He was courageous in facing death. He knew how quickly people got tired of the sick, incarcerated, infirm, and the elderly.

For years, he had silently worked hard and kept the family financially well-off. He had run a wood yard where people came to buy wood for their fireplaces and barbecue outings. He worked during the week, ran the wood business on Saturdays, prayed and read the Bible on Sundays.

People came from miles around to buy wood from Daddy B. A lot of people burned wood because it was cheaper. Air pollution was not an issue then. Men did not mind bringing in wood to keep their families warm during those days. Fireplaces were used a lot for warmth as well as for style.

The wood business was more prosperous during the winter months. Daddy B. saved all of his winter proceeds from the wood business. He was very frugal because he had lived through a depression. Rumor had it that he had money buried in large mayonnaise jars on the property.

Daddy B. had retired from work in his old age, and he had run the wood business mainly on Saturdays. Having worked hard and remaining very active had caused him to be basically physically fit. I never heard of him going to a doctor until he became ill with gout.

He rarely had even a common cold. Had he been under a doctor, gout may have been prevented or caught early enough to treat it. He wore round wire-rimmed bifocals all of his life. He never owned or wore dentures. Only when he laughed did anyone know he was edentulous.

Seeing one's parents grow old gives a feeling of pity for them. Daddy B.'s hair had completely grayed. He was stocky and bald with high front cowlicks. His mind was still quite sharp up until death. He was always compassionate and kind to everyone. He read a lot and talked little.

While writing this second publication, I had the experience of losing two sisters to death. One had suffered many embarrassing atrocities during her childhood, and she had not experienced a happy adulthood. She developed many chronic illnesses. She survived being hit by a car at age eight.

When we would get together and talk as adults, she would often say, "Sis, I am going to die." I would ask why she thought so, and she would reply, "I just know I'm going to die." I never knew whether it was a premonition or a secret wish to die, since her life had basically been an unhappy one.

As sisters, we had been separated for many years. We lived together briefly during our teen years. She did not get the chance to complete her formal education. She later completed training as a hostess. She worked in a number of households of wealthy people where she was loved and highly favored.

This sister attended the Methodist church as a young adult. Her mother-in-law and father-in-law, with whom she lived in Southern Florida, were very devout Pentecostals. They encouraged her to attend church. She gave her life to the Lord and was very devout herself for a time.

During later years, she seemed to just lose interest in life. She stated she felt condemned due to other church members' attitudes toward her. As her health failed, she declined going to church. She allowed the discouragers to hinder her church attendance.

Many people do not go to churches today because they focus on the hypocrites who are there or the imperfections of the minister and others. There will always be hypocrites and those who play with the things of God. Therefore, we must develop our own firm relationship with God. We must pray, read the word and ask the Lord to help us in our walk with him.

We must also ask the Lord to lead us to a place of worship where we can grow in the things of God. There are so many varied religious denominations until people often do not know where to begin a life with the Lord. Ask the Lord to lead you into his truths. At some point, he will do just that.

Try not to jump into the first assembled group thinking you will develop a relationship with the Lord. Listen, observe, and continue to pray for guidance in your desired walk with your maker. If you are sincere, he will see to it that you come in contact with him and his truths.

My sister knew about God from her days in the church. She and I would often sit on the porch of her high-rise and talk about Christianity. She would tell me, "Sis, I sit on this porch and look across the water, and I pray all the time."

She developed an episode of shortness of breath some time later, after many talks. She was taken to the hospital where we all thought she would be treated and then come back home. She was laughing and talking with family as she was going to the hospital. She never appeared to be in poor health, but the underlying damage was there. She exited life the next day.

The subjects of death and dying are difficult for most people. The subject is avoided as much as possible. Death is another level in the continuum of life and must be faced by all. According to scriptures, only two people were translated to Heaven by God without seeing death. These were Enoch and Elijah.

"And Enoch, [Adam's grandson] walked with God: and he was not; for God took him" Genesis 5:24. "And it came to pass, when the Lord would take up Elijah into heaven by a whirlwind that Elijah went with Elisha from Gilgal" 2 Kings 2:1. In verse 11 of 2 Kings, chapter 2, Elijah was taken up to heaven by the whirlwind.

Some would argue this to be in conflict with another scripture which says, "And as it is appointed unto men once to die, but after this the judgment" Hebrews 9:27. Remember God is sovereign and his Word will be fulfilled. He has a way to accomplish whatever he says, and he can back up his Word.

One other person was able to bargain with death. When God sent the prophet Isaiah to tell Hezekiah to get his house in order because he was going to die, Hezekiah wept and reminded God of his own works on earth. His life was extended another fifteen years. See Isaiah 38:1-22.

Like most young people, I never thought about or dwelled on the subject of death. I was almost killed three times during my youth. After I grew up, I realized God spared my life for a purpose. We experience events in life, and we may never know why. At other times, it is because we will eventually use those experiences to help others.

Many people have pleasant, uneventful lives from youth all the way through death. Some feel guilty that the people who seem to have had more dramatic lives have gotten all of the attention. I, for one, would have given everything to have had an uneventful life. It is just as okay to have an uneventful life as it is to have an event filled life.

Praying forefathers and ancestors are assets to anyone's lives. Children of praying parents do not realize the troubles, woes, and dangers they are spared from by these praying people. Having praying parents, coupled with obedience and no rebellion, can lead us to enjoyable, full, and blissful lives.

Nurses, who work in hospitals, have to deal with death and dying on a regular basis. It is important to learn how to deal with people who are experiencing death of loved ones. Their actions can run the gamut from showing open emotions or being totally overwhelmed to the point of passing out.

People live in denial of the fact that death is inevitable one day. Death is another level in the continuum of life and must be faced by all. Those who consider themselves as Christians look forward to an after life. Our belief is that one must make preparation for the after life while living on this earth. That preparation involves accepting the Lord as one's Savior. The Bible becomes the guide or road map for learning what is necessary to be prepared.

One elderly friend of mine told me she prayed for God to take her if he was not going to heal her on this earth. She was gone within about a week's time. She was a very devout woman of prayer. She had mentored me for several years in the things of God. Prior to her becoming disabled, we had shared membership in the same prayer group at our church.

People who are close to God can often petition him as to when they are ready to die. From my experience with death and dying, God has honored these people's petitions. Some patients have shown evidence that they sensed death nearby.

One night, one of our very sick hospitalized male clients began to scream out, "I see the fire. Come and get me out of this fire." He had been very unkind to all staff and constantly uttered profanities throughout his hospital stay. He passed away before the shift was over. He never got around to apologizing to any of the staff for his behavior. Some would speculate that he did not make preparation for his after life.

People, especially children, need to have an outlet for their questions and expressions of grief. Parents of dying children are usually the most difficult to console. As stated in another part of this book, losing a child hurts very deeply. People and families need closure when death occurs.

As mentioned earlier in this work, I was almost killed three times. The first time, I was almost hit by a speeding car that ran around our stopped school bus. We had no crossing guards in those days. Busing was fairly new, and we had to walk a lot of places. My older sister was hit by a car at another time, and she lived to tell about it.

The next incident occurred during a summer break. The school's recreation department bused us to the local lakes and ponds to play and swim. Few public swimming pools existed during that time. While swimming one day, I ventured into a deep hole at the bottom of the lake. I screamed and a nearby lifeguard came and rescued me.

Learning to swim as a Girl Scout in earlier years proved to be an asset at this time. It took me one whole week to overcome my fear of the water. I had a very patient swimming teacher. It was the summer just before the polio vaccine was discovered, and many children died of polio. People were kept in large cylindrical tanks called an iron lungs.

It was also common to see children walking with braces from the crippling effects of the polio. The third near-accidental-death incident occurred just days after one of Florida's notorious hurricanes. Trees and power lines had been blown down all over town. We had to return to school before all of the debris was cleared.

There was a clear path to walk, but I chose to try and climb through the fallen trees. As I was climbing through the boughs of the tree, I barely missed a power line lying on the ground. The tree had been sun dried, which apparently helped to prevent me from being killed.

God had his special angels surrounding me even then. I never bothered to tell Mother dear about these experiences and risk getting whipped. Parents sometimes think they have the best kids who will never do any wrong. While parents' backs are turned, kids try all kinds of capers.

The first deceased client I ever tended was during my first year of clinical nursing. I was sent in to remove the tubes, intravenous lines, and catheter from the client. I was also assigned to bathe this client. I felt really weird not being able to talk to the client.

For the first time in my life, I came to grips with my own mortality. I started thinking about all the teaching I had about going to heaven or the hot place. I wondered where this person went. I cleaned the person up with all the courage I could muster. Thankfully, we had a time to discuss our feelings later in class.

When I completed caring for the client, an orderly transported the body to the morgue to be picked up by the mortician. In those days, families were not allowed to come in and spend time with the corpse for closure purposes, unless special permission was granted by the doctor.

The first body I touched was that of my deceased baby sister. She had been accidentally shocked by a heater wire at age thirteen. During the funeral, I felt her face, and I was amazed at the hardness of her body. We truly go back to that from which we came.

"For dust thou art, and unto dust shalt thou return" Genesis 3:19. The night before I received the phone call about my sister's death, I had dreamed that one of my sisters would die. When I awoke, I wondered if this dream was going to be true, as many of my dreams had turned out to be in the past.

As I drove the thirteen miles to work, I was absorbed with the thought of my dream. When I arrived at work and started my routine for the day, I had an overwhelming feeling that I was going to receive a phone call connected with this dream. I received the call before our business opened.

It was a call from one of my relatives, informing me that my thirteen-year-old sister had passed away. I was given the day off to travel to be with the rest of the family. This sister had been adopted as a baby. She had just recently learned about us as her siblings.

As families do, we all sat around reminiscing the few times we had spent with this sister. Her adoptive mother told us this sister had sung and played a touching song in church the day before, which was Sunday. She had left a tearful audience as she sang and played the song, "Lord, Keep Me Day by Day."

This was another incident where I felt helpless and wished I could have done something to prevent this senseless death. I had not yet started nursing school. When I did enter nursing school, I learned that prevention is a very valuable tool for maintaining good health and preventing early deaths.

Every experience with someone's illness or death in the past served as a stimulus of interest in my studies. I studied hard and long, with the hope of being instrumental in the role of prevention. Thanks to the advent of cardiopulmonary resuscitation, lives can at least be given a chance.

Another time of caring for the dying was during my tenure at a hospital pediatrics ward. I worked alone in the isolation unit for a time. This was the time prior to successful liver transplants. Babies who were born with biliary and certain renal diseases usually died.

For many nights, I tended to these tiny, almost golden-skinned babies. Their skin and eyes were deeply yellow due to the very high content of bile pigment in their bloodstreams. With a nonfunctioning liver, there was no way their bodies could clear the system of bile and waste. The liver is the body's largest and main organ for clearing waste from the system. The kidneys, lungs, skin, and bowels are the other body-waste-eliminating systems.

Each baby had jaundiced, sunken, pathetic little eyes that stared back at me nightly from their Isolettes. Premature and ill babies were also kept in these incubator beds. As I cared for them nightly, I prayed for them and for a cure very soon. Cures have been found, and now these babies live.

During my career as a hospital nurse, death and dying were common occurrences. It was not unusual to hear a code called which summoned life savers to the distressed patient. Some of the codes were successful, and the client eventually went home. Others ended in the person passing on.

Death is an event that often leaves us feeling helpless and forced to realize our own mortality. The threat looms very real over people who suffer for years, the aged, people with terminal illnesses, and those in war zones. We are faced with the fact that we are not immortal. Those who have peace with their maker are less stressed by death.

When disasters occur, if we survive them, we are again reminded that life is not a commodity that we can hold on to if it is our time to go. People go to the hospital to relieve suffering and to get well, yet death comes while they are there. This is why we should be mindful of Psalm 90:12: "So teach us to number our days, that we may apply our hearts unto wisdom."

"Lord, make me to know mine end, and the measure of my days, what it is; that I may know how frail I am" Psalm 39:4. When we are young and strong, we feel invincible and indestructible. We don't consider the fact that we did not come into this earth to stay forever.

Those who make it to their seventieth, eightieth, ninetieth or older birth date often say they thought they would have passed away long ago. Many of their peers and contemporaries are gone. Life threatens to become lonely.

Those who have not formed a strong bond of faith and close bonds with friends and family find themselves in isolation and waiting to die. As humans, we fear the pain and uncertain hereafter of death if no concrete preparations have been made for eternity.

As it is aptly expressed in Luke 16:26: "And beside all this, between us and you there is a great gulf fixed: so that they which would pass from hence to you cannot; neither can they pass to us that would come from thence." Read Luke 16:19-31.

"So live, that when thy summons comes to join / The innumerable caravan which moves / To that mysterious realm, where each shall take / His chamber in the silent halls of death, / Thou go not, like the quarry-slave at night, / Scourged to his dungeon, but, sustained and soothed. / By an unfaltering trust, approach thy grave / Like one who wraps the drapery of his couch / About him, and lies down to pleasant dreams."

The above lines are from William Cullen Bryant's poem, "Thanatopsis." One of my high school instructors required that all of her students learn and live this poem. A peaceful death can be seen in the words of the poet.

This is what every nurse who deals with life's ending should try and help their expiring patients achieve. Clients who are facing death should be allowed to freely talk about it. Hospital chaplains are usually available when staff is not comfortable with the subject.

My most recent sister to die was nine months younger than I am. At the time of our separation from our parents, we both were age six, with me being a few months older than her. We, along with other siblings, were placed into different homes in different locations. This sister experienced many atrocities as well as an abusive marriage.

This sister also developed a lot of chronic illnesses, including cardiovascular problems. She had stents applied in her heart for blockages along the way. She too did not complete her early education. As an adult, she went back to school, and then she completed a career in the medical profession. She worked many years while she reared her family.

She was very devout. She sang and preached as a missionary in the churches in many Northern cities. She also taught her five children the way of the Lord. Three of them preceded her in death in their young adult years. She said that when her children died, she would have lost it had she not been anchored in the Lord.

This sister flew down to be at our oldest sister's burial. When she landed at the international airport, a police officer called me to come and get her because she was ill. I responded. Before I could reach the airport I received another call from the officer requesting that I meet my sister in the city's hospital emergency room.

When I reached the emergency room, my sister was lying on a cardiac bed in one of the patient areas of the emergency room. Her cardiac status was being monitored. She had been complaining of chest pains on the trip, and the airline staff and the officers did not want to take a chance on her getting worse.

I phoned my sister's oldest daughter back up North. My niece informed me that her mom probably hadn't taken her medications nor eaten anything all day; this was probably the reason for the episode. My niece was right. In her haste to get to our other sister's funeral, my sister had left her medications in her luggage.

She signed herself out from the hospital AMA (against medical advice). She insisted that she had not come this far to miss seeing her sister for the last time. We ceased trying to convince her to stay in the hospital. Her mind was made up. We knew she needed the closure. Those two siblings had spent more time together than the rest of us.

We made sure she rested and got her medications and her meals. I sensed that she was very ill, but she was trying to be stoic. She refused to return to the hospital, saying she would see her own doctor back home. We honored her wishes. She made it to the funeral and got the closure she desperately desired and needed.

My sister went back to her home two days later. Less than two months later, another niece called to say that one of my sisters had passed away. We have another sister who has been ill for several years, and I feared it was her. This sister had been given five years to live twenty years ago.

She is alive, and doing quite well, despite the diagnosis twenty years ago. She was advised to go on dialysis some years ago. She refused dialysis and is still alive. She and I talk sometimes daily or at least weekly by phone. She loves to go fishing and does so regularly. She is indeed a miracle. Although we live several thousand miles apart, I recently visited her. I also recently traveled and spent time with this sister.

I was bombarded with thoughts of how fleeting life is and how we have to cherish every moment we have with our loved ones. The two sisters who had suffered so much in life were now gone from their earthly sufferings. My faith sustained me. I sensed this was my last encounter with this sister. I was right.

This second sister that passed away had told me she and her son-in-law planned to conduct a huge yard sale upon her return home. My niece said my sister and the son-in-law had gotten everything together for the sale. My sister slipped away just prior to the event. There was no struggle. She just slept away.

The yard sale and the people she had planned to meet would also never see her again. Her seat at the fishing pond has been vacated forever. "He shall no more return to his house, neither shall his place know him any more" Job 7:10.

She had the stents placed in her heart approximately ten years ago. I could not help but feel that the stress of the trip perhaps hastened her demise. By pressing her way to our older sister's funeral, she shortened her own life. She did not care whether she lived; she just wanted to see her sister one more time.

These two sisters had been together all of their lives, except for the brief time my older sister and I had been in the same home. They had experienced the abuses by the same people, dropped out of school, and then pursued their careers in later years.

This sister and I got a chance to fellowship and enjoy each other's company before returning to our separate destinations. We talked a lot about what happened to us over the years as adults. We had intended to discuss another traumatic event in her life, but we never got around to it.

That is the situation with death. Whatever we fail to say to someone on this side of eternity has to be left unsaid. There is just no way to fix any undone business we might have had with them. Losing two sisters back to back was a challenge that only a God relationship can mend.

For weeks, I headed to the phone to call them, only to remember that they were no longer on this earth. I could not reach across the fixed gulf to talk to neither one of them. The finality of their being gone has finally set in. We'll never giggle together again on this earth.

Retirement

This section will begin with an admonishment to new nurses and nurses who change jobs frequently. Nothing is more disconcerting to anyone who has worked for years than finding oneself retired without certain provisions. Visions of retirement bring up lifelong dreams of travel and generally enjoying life.

New nurses need to think about savings and investing. The excitement of suddenly earning large amounts of money may cause you to be tempted to buy the latest luxury car, the biggest home you can find, a large closet of the most fashionable clothes and all kinds of nice trinkets.

Truth is, all of those things depreciate. You may live a life of ease with no lack for years. If you have not prepared for retirement, the life of no lack will quickly turn into a life of poverty. With the nation's social security system threatened and retirement programs going belly up, one needs to seriously look at alternative retirement options.

Find a reputable financial planning institution and discuss your options. Keep your own individual retirement account (IRA). Learn to do more than one career in life. While nursing is a great career, some situations may render you unable to work as a nurse.

Employers tend to look among the young for workers. They are not interested in filling their work places with the aged or infirm. Music and cosmetology have been wonderful alternative money-making skills for me. Eight-to-five jobs have a way of ending when a worker is unable to keep up.

If you have other talents and skills, develop them early in your working years. If you've had ideas to invent something or to do something that brings in income, carry them along with any career. Not only will it help in your present job, it may end up being your retirement income.

Retirement is a wonderful time of feeling freedom such as you may have never felt it. There are no time clocks to punch, no unexpected meetings to attend while you place your most pressing assignments on hold, and no traffic nightmares morning and afternoon to endure getting to and from the job.

Safety net savings can get depleted very fast in today's economy. Whatever you do, don't resort to credit cards to take up the slack in your finances. That is a no-brainer. Resist the urge to please everyone by spending money on them. If they are true family and friends, they won't expect it.

The benefits of the tithe are discussed in my first book *Natural Bread Is Not Enough*. Do not become stingy, but use wisdom in your finances. Malachi chapter 3 of the Old Testament gives the benefits of the tithe. Supporting God's work brings blessings.

Finally, avoid job hopping. If you want to try different areas of nursing before settling for one, join an institution that has such a program or do some volunteer work. Keep abreast of what's happening in nursing and keep up your skills. Get plenty of ICU and emergency room skills.

Early in the year of 1992, I attended an evangelistic convention in the Western United States. This was a prophetic conference called "Let the Healing Begin." Ministers and conference attendees were prophetically warned as to what to expect of the economy in the coming decade.

People were warned to pay off their homes, cars, and credit card accounts. The Lord showed the host minister the future of the economy, and he was instructed to warn conference attendees. My own pastor held a conference some years ago, and he gave the same prophecies to warn the people.

People who heeded the warnings did not lose their homes when mortgage companies went belly up. Those who obeyed and were frugal with their finances are faring well in today's economy. Those who have gotten rid of the credit card debts are being spared the exorbitant interest rates.

From my perspective as a retired person, I would continue to warn nurses and others that are still in the job market to save and to invest wisely. "Be thou diligent to know the state of thy flocks, and look well to thy herds. For riches are not for ever" Proverbs 27:23-24. Pay off all debts!

Retirement can be a very fast exit out of the land of the living. All of that left over energy from the day-to-day grind needs to be put to constructive use. Suddenly there is liberty to do all those projects you have thrown on the back burner for years. There's time for extensive travel and other pursuits.

Discipline was never more important than it is now. It is easy to lounge around all day watching television, and sleeping in every day. Suddenly every day is a weekend. A College professor of mine was nearing retirement. His entire song was "I'm going to sit on the patio every day and sip drinks when I retire."

His name appeared in the obituary section of the paper pretty soon after his retirement. While the rest, relaxation, and reduced stress are great, retirees need to use time wisely. Keep occupied with constructive and productive activities. Keep dreaming. Spend time in meditation and refreshing your spirit.

There are times when you need to learn to say no, if you haven't already. Some people will start making their own schedule and agenda of commitments for you. Some well-meaning friends and neighbors think you need something to fill all those extra hours. Be selective as to what you get into.

Help when and where you can without getting yourself into bondage. When I first retired, I was bombarded with assignments from every direction by people who think retirees are excellent candidates for filling in empty spaces. Be available for helping with just causes, not just empty spaces.

The past forty-five years spent in nursing have been an adventure as well as a thrill. I have witnessed many lives enter the world and seen many lives ebb away from the earth. I have witnessed the highs and the lows with all types of people and families. The years have been both a blessing and a joy.

When I retired, many of my friends made it a true time of rejoicing. They showered me with finances, costly gifts, and a scrumptious dinner at my favorite restaurant. I actually retired twice. The opportunity presented itself to work several hours a week in a temporary position, and I took it.

Retirement, marriage, childbirth, divorce, and death of loved ones are some of the most stressful times in our lives. These require an adjustment period. Retirement, aside from having its pleasant side, is a time of some stress. One has to adjust to a different life style along with advancing age.

Something has to replace those long hours of being in the public and commuting to and from work. Reading, praying and meditating, volunteering, and playing the piano consume a lot of my time. Writing consumes another block of time. Additional time is spent with friends and family.

Church life, choir rehearsals, benevolent activities, and public prayer all consume another portion of my life. There are still hours that are not taken which I carefully choose to fill. One finds that life is not about filling in hours, but about making sure those hours are filled with quality moments.

For people who have carved out their lives away from the core family, this can be a time of deciding—do I go to live around family and familiar friends, or do I make the best of life where I live now? I have several friends who are removed from the core body of their families.

They desire to return to their families, but the economy has rendered them unable to relocate and make the transition. Since I knew my likelihood of relocating was remote, I asked the Lord to surround me with family. I solicited the prayers of my pastor and others who prayed.

I located family members that I never knew were here. They have extended family members, which make it quite a large family. Another niece and her husband, her daughter and two granddaughters, along with my niece's three sons also moved here as a direct result of the prayers.

While the phone is a wonderful tool for staying connected with family, it is not like being there. As one ages, being around good family and friends becomes very important. We realize that we are interdependent upon each other for fellowship. An old song says, "No man is an island."

Over the years, I have met young people who could not wait to get away from core family so they could do their own thing. Like the young birds leaving the nest and trying to fly for the first time, they flit off somewhere and connect with the rest of the world. Wandering too far from family has its down side.

There are times when the Lord will lead people to go to live in a certain place. He will orchestrate the events of your life when he is the one who leads you to live in a place. Things will fall in place like clockwork. He will place whom he wants in your life. Keep in touch with family no matter where you go.

There are times when circumstances take people to places they thought they would never live. The military husband may take his wife far away from her core family or vice versa. Marriage may also cause people to move far away from their families.

At other times, people may travel to towns where they can find better jobs, or they may have been transferred to another city by their job. Whatever the case, retirement and aging may make one consider home again. If there was ever a core family and home, there is no place like it.

Some years ago, I selected a city in Central Florida where I had planned to move upon retirement. I purchased a large three-bedroom, two-bath home. The home was a beautiful cinder-block, brick-front house with a fairly large-fenced yard. Pastel-yellow appliances filled the very large kitchen.

This was going to be my dream retirement home. The home was worth around two hundred thousand dollars, but because of the surroundings, it sold for thirty two thousand dollars. It never occurred to me to inquire as to why the man was really selling so cheaply.

The owner had grown up near me. He was a child during the time I was a teen. I felt like he was giving me a break because he knew me. Instead he was fleeing because of a vendetta the occupants of the house had with him. He had forced them out by selling the house out from under them.

In addition to the vendetta, most of the people on the street were living in nice large homes that had been let out to HUD and Section A. Most of the owners had gone up North to work and had let their homes out to rent. My home was also two streets over from a crime-infested project development.

There was a time when some Southerners moved up North to high-paying jobs, made big money, saved it, paid off their homes, cars, etc., down South, and eventually moved back with finances to live a good life. This was the case on this street.

Not knowing all of this, I came along and bought the house. Since I worked the night shift, I rarely saw my neighbors. One young man who was getting ready to go away to College confided in me. He told me this was the type of neighborhood where people were very jealous of each other.

He advised me not to get my lawn mowed and to let my property run down a little. He said, "Otherwise they will make it bad for you here." I could not understand what he was talking about. He soon left for College, and I forgot about him and the warning. I kept my property in good shape.

Eventually, someone started dumping their garbage in my yard. Every morning while I was sleeping after I had worked all night, there was new garbage. I would stay up to see if I could catch them, but I never could do so. I inquired among the neighbors and no one saw anything, they said.

Another morning, I ran over some brown bags that were left in the road where I had to turn into my car port. I heard the crunching sounds as I drove into my yard. I went to bed and when I woke up, all four of my tires were flat. After that, someone started breaking into my house. They broke in twice.

The Lord had shown me someone was going to break in the first time, so I got a house dog. One day, someone poisoned the dog while he was out in the yard and broke in a second time. On another occasion, someone placed a baby rattlesnake in my front screen door and pushed the screen shut.

After having worked all night, I had spent the day taking care of important business. I had not had any sleep, so I came home at dusk to get a nap before going to my usual night shift. As I opened the door, I saw the snake. I called a neighbor, who came over with his hoe and killed the snake.

Finally, I set out to find out who was doing all of this mischief and why. I learned that the people that had a vendetta with the home seller were venting their frustrations on me. One young lady told me exactly who was doing the acts. I prayed for them and sold the property, and then I moved away.

That was the end of the retirement house. I had not consulted the Lord about this house. It was a painful lesson about not looking a gift horse in the mouth from the story of the Trojan horse. I forgave the people who did the mischief without knowing them or them ever knowing I had forgiven them.

When we are innocently wronged by others, the results of their acts are going to come back to them. That is why we need to be sure we treat each other with love and respect. Those who insist on being bad people are best left alone as we move on.

Retirement is a time of reflecting on our years and what we have done with those years. Those who are blessed to retire and live any length of time should count it as a blessing. I have worked with coworkers who were ill. They struggled to make it to retirement, but they died within days or months before retirement.

One coworker, who was younger than me, was sitting in a staff meeting one day. She had appeared to be the picture of health. I learned that she died while the staff meeting was in progress. I had recently fellowshipped with her. Since she was younger than me, I never dreamed I wouldn't see her again.

Retirement can be a time of new beginnings. Some retirees embark upon another career. Youth and good health with retirement are wonderful assets. It has been wonderful still being young enough to enjoy the other things that I was blessed to learn during my earlier years.

Prayer and spiritual refreshing continues to be the one thing that keeps me going during my retirement. Playing or just listening to praise music at any hour is a great refresher if and when I am tempted to worry about the fact that I am no longer on the job. They are doing just fine without me.

CONCLUSION

There are people who have within them the desire to relieve the sick and suffering of others. There are also those who desire to see a healthier population and to assist in procedures that foster good health. There are many careers within the health field that may satisfy these desires.

The medical career gamut extends from physicians to medical volunteers. A nursing career was my choice to satisfy this desire to help the sick and the suffering as well as myself. I have heard people say, "I would like to be a nurse, but I cannot stand the sight of blood." There are other choices these days than being a nurse or a doctor.

A visit to a local medical center or hospital will allow one to see all types of medical personnel. Let's begin with the paramedics who may have brought the patient to the hospital. This is a medical career. You will do a lot of what people do in hospitals. The person's medical record was initiated by the paramedics.

There is also a medical records department at the hospital and at every medical institution. Those who want to be near the arena of action but not have all of the blood exposure may choose a career in medical records. Many careers are seen along the path to hospital admission and within the institution itself.

Paramedics try and stabilize the patients before taking them to the hospital. They assess the vital signs such as blood pressure, temperature, respiration rate, and pulse. Each of these vital signs can give a clue to what is going on in the patient's body.

Intravenous (IV) fluids are usually started on the patient. These fluids provide necessary hydration. The IV itself provides a port of entry for medications, blood, or whatever else the body needs at this time. In the past, venipuncture was done only by doctors, nurses, and paramedics.

Nowadays, there is an entire profession devoted to the practice of phlebotomy. The phlebotomist is highly skilled and trained to start intravenous fluids and to perform other procedures where vein or artery entry is necessary. The phlebotomist is a most welcomed member of the medical team.

A myriad of health workers now make up the medical team. There are therapists of every type. These workers are summoned as needed and may continue to see the patient throughout his hospital stay. Clerical staff is always needed to record events and medical information about the client.

Security workers are becoming more vital in medical areas. Human traffic control and safety of patients and staff are more of a consideration now than in years past. Parking areas are considered safer when security is present. The criminal element is more prolific now than in past years.

Nursing is a profession that allows nurses and medical personnel to meet and see clients at their most vulnerable moments. The lady who just simply cannot step out into public without her makeup is suddenly seen without makeup. She perhaps was too ill to care about makeup.

Then there is the person who may have been in a tragic auto accident. His rescue may have depended on being removed from his auto via the Jaws of Life. His clothing may have been cut from him. The hospital gown he was required to don further exposed him and left him with little dignity.

A life and death situation in which we may find ourselves may force us to display primitive behavior. A mom may be thrown into the depths of grief by the sudden knowledge of her child being killed. At that moment, she is not concerned with appearances.

When I was told of my own fetal losses, I cried bitterly and did not care who heard or saw me. In these instances, tact and discretion need to be present. Compassion and empathy need to be real. We must have the utmost of respect for those in our care who for whatever reason find themselves vulnerable.

In training, we were taught that hearing is the last sense to leave the body prior to death. It has been documented that comatose people have heard entire conversations uttered over them. People who had near death experiences have repeated what they heard spoken while they were in surgery.

These people were under anesthesia, yet they could repeat every word each person had said. Others were comatose for months, yet they could remember statements uttered by caregivers. Just because someone is not responding to you does not mean they are not hearing what you are saying.

As a passenger on an airplane that was falling some years ago, all I cared about was how I would fare in the afterlife that I had been taught about all my life. That one experience has caused me to be mindful of how I treat others. We were all on the verge of displaying our raw emotions.

Having spent forty-five years in some medical capacity has allowed me to come to grips with the fact that none of us is better than the other. Some of us are materially better off than others, and some perhaps are deemed better looking than others. But at the end of the day, we are all still human beings.

When we are alone in an unfamiliar city or country, without our pocketful of identification, no one knows or cares who we happen to be. "Naked came I out of my mother's womb, and naked shall I return thither: the Lord gave, and the Lord hath taken away" Job 1:21.

These are the words uttered by the biblical patriarch Job when he went through bitter trials of his faith in God. The medical profession is a very humbling position. It forces one to swallow pride and admit that we are all created equally by one creator. Man assigns his own brand of equality to others.

Nursing is a rewarding profession to those who love it. It is also a profession where one gives of himself/herself continuously. It can lend itself quickly to burnout if the practitioners do not learn to separate the job from their personal lives.

At first, it was very difficult for me to separate job from self. As time went by and the wear and tear was felt, I learned to empathize or sympathize, do what I could do, and move on. No one can be all things to all people at all times. Helping one to help himself is far better than enabling him.

It has been my experience with enabling people is that if they are allowed to do so, they attach themselves to you and cripple themselves as well as you. Some of them see you as a permanent supplier of all of their needs, especially when they get in trouble. I acquired the name "Super Nurse" at one time while trying to meet everyone's needs.

Growing up in the midst of plenty made me want to embrace every disadvantaged person and meet all of their needs. Channeling people's energies into self-help is more beneficial. While the majority of clients have been independent, a few have attempted to become enablers.

By the time a nurse or doctor goes through the rotation of specialties, they have an idea of the area in which they'd like to practice. Some specialties are far more active than others. Areas such as the intensive care units and emergency room and trauma units tend to be the most active areas.

Medical, surgical, obstetrical, pediatric, and psychiatric nursing can be very active at times. This requires that staff be extremely vigilant at all times. Public health also requires vigilance, but it is an area where more time can be spent on one entity. Every moment is not crisis filled.

Some staff members thrive on the constant excitement and the adrenaline pumping pace of the ER, the ICU, and the trauma units. Other staff members prefer the slower-paced units. A nurse can find her niche because there are so many areas from which to choose.

At one point, I was given the opportunity to fly in a helicopter to pick up babies from smaller hospitals. They were brought into the teaching hospital to receive more acute care. I thought I would love this type of nursing. I could not wait to get started. When the starting day arrived, we boarded the aircraft.

We flew off on our mission. I was impressed with the idea of constantly flying to get these babies and participating in their care in our hospital. We must have gotten the most dilapidated helicopter there was on the first day. It rattled and shook and threatened to crash during the entire trip.

The noise level almost deafened me. One trip convinced me that I could not do this every day. Care for the babies? Yes. Fly to get them? No. Had I been warned about the helicopter, I might have tried to adjust. After the first trip, I abandoned the aviation part of nursing. Aviation was exciting, but not for me.

FINALE

Forty-five years for me have come and gone. They were only as yesterday. Time has a way of moving on whether we move with it or not. While I accomplished some things, I could have accomplished far more had I not wasted time and made wiser decisions. All of us waste time which can never be recaptured.

There were the years of pursuing dreams that were never meant to be. That is why the word says, "But seek ye first the kingdom of God, and his righteousness; and all these things shall be added unto you" Matthew 6:33. When we put our maker first in everything, we experience success in all things.

Unfortunately, a lot of us only think of our maker when we are in trouble. When there is a national crisis, people find the time to pray and observe moments of silence. Prayer is our last resort when it should be our first. Prayer occupies center stage until our crises are over.

It has been interesting to see people, events, as well as the profession evolve over time. Nursing wearing apparel is one of the most prominent changes to behold. Forty-five years ago, nurses and medical people all donned white uniforms daily for work.

Rarely do we see a predominance of white uniforms in any medical institution anymore. Occasionally, a church will host some affair where women wear all-white attire, but few, especially the younger staff, are familiar with the practice. Scrubs are seen everywhere nowadays.

Twenty-first-century strolls down the hospital halls reveal many different colors of scrub suits being worn. Each department is identified by a different color scrub suit. Some staff members wear casual clothing under a white or pastel lab jacket. There is no way to quickly spot nurses these days.

There are more and varied departments doing different services for clients now. In the past, some hospitals had no other disciplines except nursing. Along with everything else, nurses conducted respiratory therapy. Nurses were often given tasks no one else desired or floated anywhere to meet staffing quotas.

It is my hope that those who read this forty-five-year account of some of my life and career will be inspired to make wise use of your time and resolve to choose a career that you love. Better still, embrace and develop those God-given talents which are already within you.

Hopefully, that career will be nursing or some area of the medical profession. Health care will always be necessary. Someone needs to be prepared and available to care for the health needs of all of us. Choose an area where going to the job daily will be pleasurable.

Many nurses have worked in the profession far more years than I have, and I believe their accounts perhaps are far more exciting and more interesting. I could not have told the story without mentioning the life events that spurred me along. Here's to hoping you enjoyed my account.

Guard your health

Never have I seen in all of my years such a feverish conquest for good health. Exercise studios and clubs are proliferating, television shows are preoccupied with health programs, and many people are obsessed with acquiring a sleek body.

While some in the clothing industry are trying to constantly come up with attractive attire for the obese, others are trying to design clothing that give a slimming appearance to bulky bodies. While all of these are great efforts, there are many health-enhancing activities we can adopt on a daily basis.

Listening to the gospel stations on Sunday mornings before church service was once a popular Afro-American tradition. Gospel music was often sung between sermons by various preachers. Some of the faith healers also got in on the programming.

There was one particular faith healer who would instruct the radio audience to place a large glass of water atop the radio during the program. Then the healer would tell the people to drink the large glass of water after he had prayed over it.

HYDRATE YOUR BODY

A lot of people were suffering from various conditions due to lack of proper hydration. Some drank sodas mainly instead of drinking water. When they drank the large glass of water, they were amazed at how much better they felt. People attributed their good feeling to the faith healer. While prayer helped, their body had just gotten the water it desperately needed.

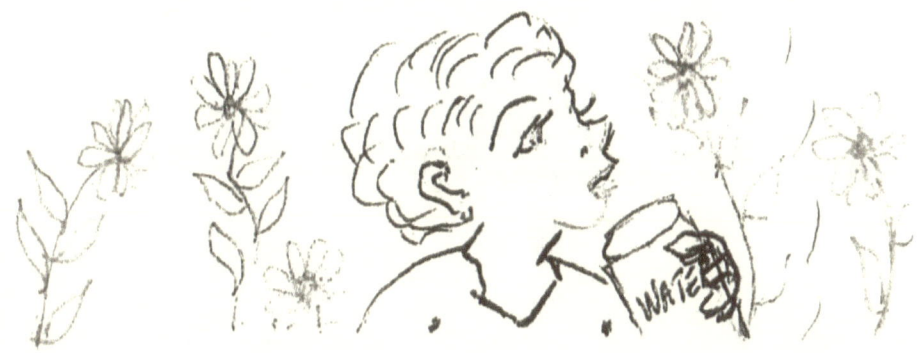

Like a flower garden, this body must have water to survive. Water is needed in the body as a temperature regulator, lubricant, and a cleanser to take away waste material. It is also needed for construction of body cells and acts as a solvent in the breaking down of food for the body to use.

Various resources differ on what is adequate water intake. Other resources say we get part of our water intake from the foods we eat. Water intake varies with age, activity, and caloric intake. Some resources recommend six eight-ounce glasses per day as adequate water intake for adults.

GET ADEQUATE REST AND SLEEP

Lack of sleep and rest can lead to disorientation, unnecessary weight gain, and crankiness. Drivers who nod off and sleep while on the highway pose threats to others on the roadways. The body needs time to rejuvenate itself.

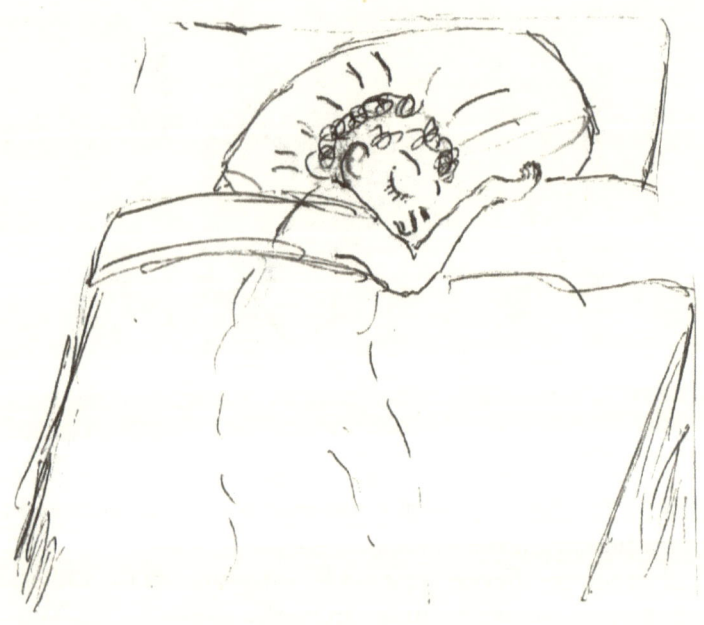

"I will both lay me down in peace, and sleep: for thou, Lord, only makest me dwell in safety" Psalm 4:8.

WASH HANDS FREQUENTLY

One of the most powerful offensive weapons against diseases and illnesses is hand washing. Hand sanitizers are now strategically placed in many public places. In the absence of soap and water, hand sanitizers are good substitutes.

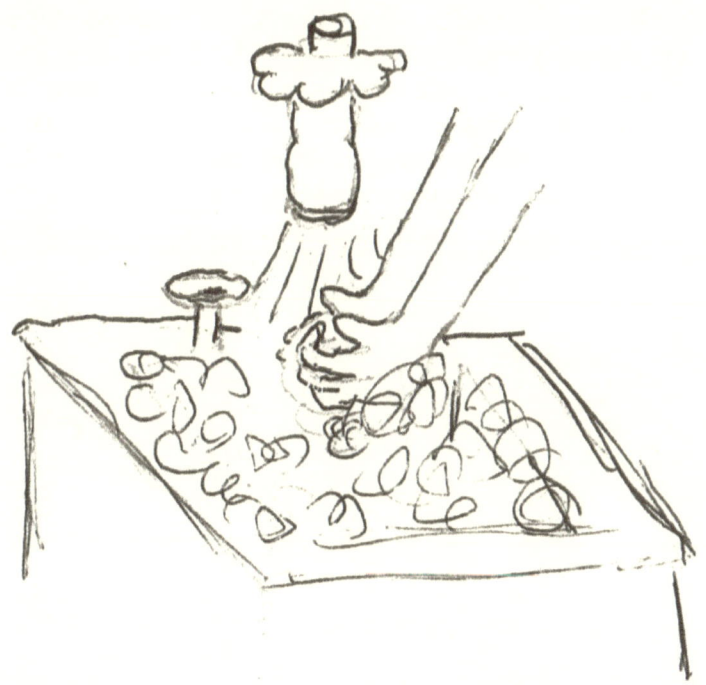

Medical personnel are taught glove technique and universal precautions for handling contaminated material.

GET SCHEDULED
IMMUNIZATIONS ON TIME

Research supports the fact that immunizations have been valuable in eliminating many of the dreaded diseases. Diseases such as tetanus, whooping cough, diphtheria, polio, and smallpox that killed many people, especially children, are now rarely heard about.

Prior to that time, polio victims were put on display in large cylindrical tanks in public places. I first saw one of these at the Lake County fair. As kids, we gawked and were amazed at these large noisy tanks. Soon the polio vaccine was invented, and these tanks disappeared.

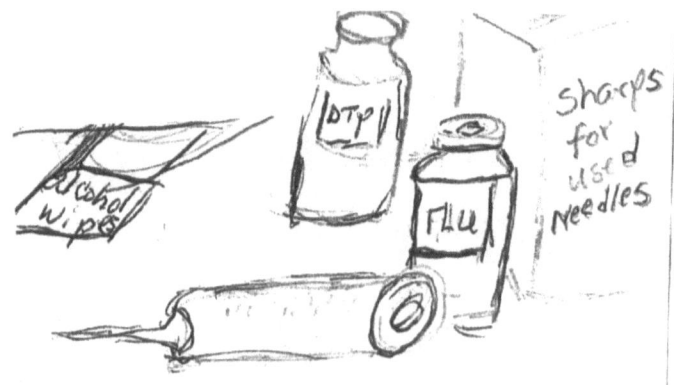

Before traveling abroad, check with your local health department to see if you will need immunizations for the areas to which you will travel. These diseases can be contracted abroad if you are not immunized. Some countries do not have the same immunization standards found in the USA.

OBSERVE QUIET TIMES

Meditation, reflection, and prayer are great refreshers. When an appliance is allowed to burn around the clock, it quickly burns out. A body that is forced to go continuously without quiet time soon burns out. Our spirits as well as our bodies benefit greatly from constant renewal.

One winter, my heat failed to function in the middle of the night. I turned on the oven unit in an effort to keep my home warm until the next day. The stress of burning the unit caused it to burn out quicker because it wasn't designed to burn continuously. Neither are our bodies and minds designed for 24/7 wear.

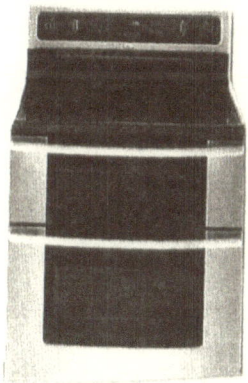

It is suggested that a regular time be set aside daily for refreshing of our mind and our spirit. Reading the word is also a great refresher. It helps to fill our spirit, as explained in my first book. Spiritual refreshing seems to increase creativity and productivity.

FRESH AIR AND SUNSHINE ARE ESSENTIAL TO GOOD HEALTH

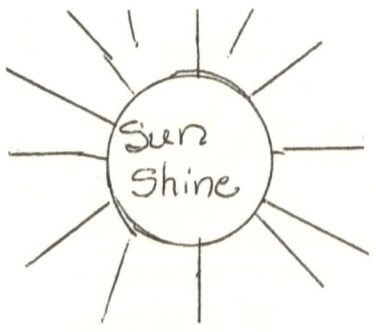

Activity and exercise do a body good.

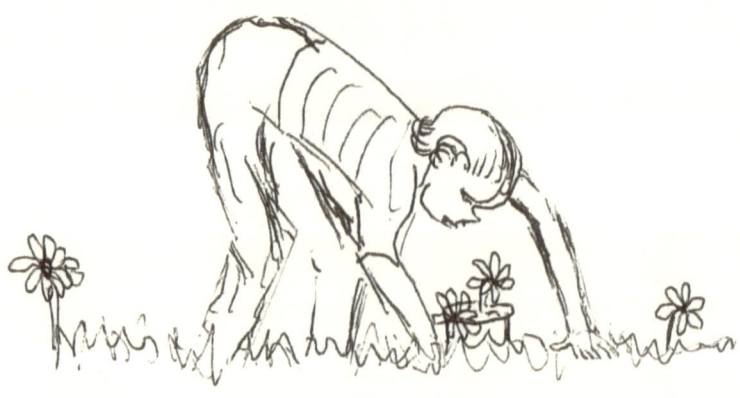

EAT HEALTHY FOODS. ENJOY MEALS WITH FAMILY AND FRIENDS WHEN POSSIBLE.

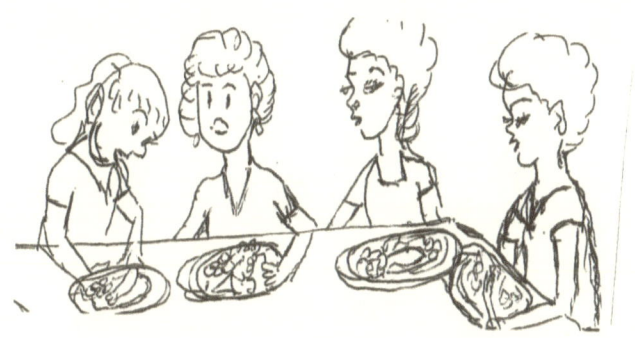

Avoid binge eating and pigging out.

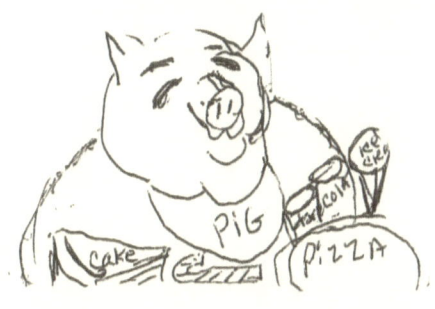

REFERENCES

Benenson, Abram S. *Control of Communicable Diseases in Man.* New York: American Public Health Association, 1970.

Dake, Finis Jennings. *The Dake Annotated Reference Bible.* King James Version. Lawrenceville, Georgia: Dake Publishing, 1991.

D'Antonio, Patricia. *American Nursing: A History of Knowledge, Authority, and the Meaning of Work.* Baltimore: The Johns Hopkins Press, 2010.

Donahue, Patricia. *Nursing, the Finest Art: An Illustrated History.* St. Louis Missouri: C. V. Mosby Company, 1985.

Henry, Matthew. *The Matthew Henry Commentary.* Grand Rapids: Zondervan Publishing House. 1981.

McGhee, J. Vernon. *Through the Bible: Genesis through Deuteronomy.* Nashville: Thomas Nelson Publishers, 1981.

Olmoguez, Violeta. *How to Write and Assemble Your Own Book.* Jacksonville: Zoë University.

Olmoguez, Violeta. *Domestic Violence: Open Up the Truth.* Jacksonville: Zoë University.

Olmoguez, Violeta. *A Handbook of Domestic Violence for Pastor, Ministers.* Jacksonville: Zoë University.

Small, Hugh. *Florence Nightingale: Avenging Angel.* New York: St. Martin's Press, 1999.

Smith, William. *Smith's Bible Dictionary.* Atlanta: Thomas Nelson Publishers, 1986.

Strong, James. *The New Strong's Concordance of the Bible.* Nashville: Thomas Nelson Publishers, 1985.

www.ingramcontent.com/pod-product-compliance
Lightning Source LLC
Chambersburg PA
CBHW032018170526

45157CB00002B/750